I0396975

Intermittent Fasting For Women 101:

A 2 Manuscript Book on the Ketogenic Diet and Intermittent Fasting: Complete Keto Meal Plan Guide For Dramatic Weight Loss

Minerva Publishing Services & Company

Ketogenic Diet and Intermittent Fasting:
The Complete Guide for Beginners Including Keto Snack Recipes, Meal Prep, and Mental Clarity

Minerva Publishing Services & Company

KETOGENIC DIET AND INTERMITTENT FASTING

The Complete Guide for Beginners

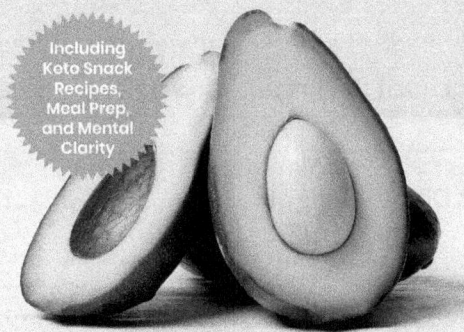

Including Keto Snack Recipes, Meal Prep, and Mental Clarity

MINERVA P.S. & CO

MINERVA PUBLISHING SERVICES & COMPANY

Table of Contents

Introduction

The ketogenic diet saves all. It has saved many individuals around the world including myself. Everyone knows about diabetes. People usually think that someone who gets diabetes deserves it because they eat foods such as McDonald's or Wendy's. The blame isn't on them. If there is a blame to diabetes it is to the whole entire education system on it.

Medicine has it all wrong and some doctors now are trying to educate people on what to do. Diabetes is serious and it kills more people than AIDS and breast cancer combined. The ADA or the American Diabetes Association says that 130 people every 24 hours develop kidney failure due to diabetes. We cannot cure diabetes but we can reverse it meaning that through diet and exercise we can stay away from diabetes.

In society, we have been taught to eat mostly carbohydrates. This has caused humans to achieve brilliant records in athletics such as faster mile times or faster swimming records. This is great but it also has caused individuals to develop diabetes.

What is diabetes? Diabetes Type II is the inability to absorb carbohydrates resulting in the glucose sugar levels to reach numbers high above normal levels. This increase in sugar is because our friend insulin isn't able to let glucose enter our cells properly.

Okay now quick science 101 intro! Insulin is a hormone that is released from the pancreas by beta cells. Insulin's main job is to allow more glucose transport proteins on the membrane of a cell. That is all insulin does. The increase in glucose transport proteins allows more glucose from the blood to be transported to the cell. Now when our body detects that glucose isn't going to the cell, all it does is increase the secretion of insulin. This will result in high insulin levels and a high glucose level in the blood because it is not able to go into the cell. So, what do we call high insulin levels and high blood sugar? It's Diabetes!

Okay so why talk so much about diabetes. About 70 percent of the USA cannot synthesize and absorb glucose efficiently. This means that people need to change the way they eat or else a lot more people will start dying from diabetes. There are three types of people when it comes to carbohydrates and dieting. The three types are insulin sensitive, insulin resistant, and the lucky ones. The lucky ones are people who don't have any issue with the transportation of glucose into the cell. The insulin resistant ones are people who cannot get glucose into the cell at all. The insulin sensitive ones are people who can get some glucose into cells but only a little bit. This book is for the insulin resistant and sensitive ones.

The only way to know if you are insulin resistant or insulin sensitive is by diet and checking your blood sugar levels every day. If your doctor told you that you have prediabetes because your A1C is at 5.7% or above then you need to listen up. An A1C is a test that measures blood glucose levels over the past 3 months. This test just measures what we talked about. The goal is to have an A1C below 5.7%. We can do this by eating less carbohydrates or even eating no carbohydrates at all.

Glucose is important for the body and the brain but we do not need to consume it because our body makes it. We have all heard of essential amino acids and essential fatty acids. There is no such thing as an essential carbohydrate. I just need to say that because so many people say we need carbohydrates but they know nothing of how the human digestion system works.

I've spent 4 years studying at Temple University and I see people online delivering false information about nutrition.

I have one more thing to say before I dive into what this book is mainly about. The ADA tells doctors to tell their patients with prediabetes to just simply reduce carbohydrate intake and eat a healthier diet. This will not solve the issue at hand. Then if the patient has diabetes the doctor is supposed to give you insulin injections that only work if you eat carbohydrates. If you don't eat carbohydrates with the medicine it will cause trauma to your gastrointestinal tract or in order words an upset stomach.

I hope you can see this cycle of carbohydrates being thrown around as if it wasn't the problem. The problem is carbohydrate toxicity in the body and we must simply reverse our body into eating fats and proteins. This will save you around 2,000 dollars' worth of medicine a year. It could save our economy billions of dollars spent on medicine for diabetes. I believe that by publishing books like this we can take the right steps into a more healthy and knowledgeable country.

This book, *Ketogenic Diet and Intermittent Fasting: The Complete Guide for Beginners Including Keto Snack Recipes, Meal Prep, and Mental Clarity,* contains recipes that can be made for breakfast, lunch, dinner, or as a dessert. Each meal grouping contains 14 recipes. All you have to do is choose one for breakfast, another for lunch, and another for dinner. There are also 7 delectable recipes for dessert. These Ketogenic meals will help you lose weight by reducing the number of carbs consumed on a daily basis. We provide all the macros and nutritional information for each recipe.

The only thing we didn't provide was a picture of the meals. We are currently working with photographers and photos will be added to the next edition.

On a last note, we try to introduce beginners to the Ketogenic diet by giving a brief overview of what this diet is all about and how it works in your body. You will also learn some of the planning techniques you should use, as well as the benefits of the Ketogenic diet. Losing weight and improving your health must start in your mind, and we include a chapter on some of the steps you can take to stay motivated throughout the journey. Watch out for some success tips for beginners at the end of the book.

There is also a section about intermittent fasting and how you can use that to your advantage, if you want to take your weight loss to the next level.

Enjoy the book, as well as the dishes!

Chapter 1:

Overview of the Ketogenic Diet

The Ketogenic diet is simply a diet that incorporates consumption of very little carbohydrates, moderate quantities of protein, and high quantities of fat. This may seem strange to someone who wants to lose fat from their body, but as we explain below fat isn't the enemy; carbs are!

How Does the Ketogenic Diet Work?

If you look at your current diet, you will realize that it is made up of mostly carbs and sugars. When you eat a lot of carbohydrates, your body breaks it down to form glucose, which is used for energy production. When glucose is produced, insulin is also produced in order to transport the glucose to every body organ. However, it also does something else: in case there is already enough glucose in the bloodstream, the insulin starts storing the excess glucose in the form of fat to be used later as an energy source.

So what happens if the person is always consuming excess carbs as an energy source? More fat is stored around their body but it is never given the opportunity to be used as an energy source! This results in weight gain.

The Ketogenic diet does the opposite of your regular diet. It recommends consumption of foods high in the good kind of fats so that your body no longer has to rely on glucose from carbs as an energy source. The goal is to teach your body to break down fats to produce energy, and with time, your body will learn to break down its own excess fatty tissue to provide energy.

Ketogenic Metabolism

It is important to understand the metabolic changes that occur when you transition from glucose-burning to fat-burning. Without carbohydrates to provide glucose, the body resorts to breaking down fats into Free Fatty Acids (FFAs), which can be used by the body's organs as fuel. The only exceptions are the brain and nervous system.

These FFAs are broken down in the liver to produce *ketones*, which are the fuel source that the brain and nervous system can use for energy. When these ketones fill the bloodstream, the body is said to be in a state of *ketosis*, which is similar to what happens during starvation. The body is simply using up these ketones to keep the body nourished and energetic.

There is no need to fear ketosis since it is just mimicking starvation but without the harmful effects. A Ketogenic diet will help your body rely on fats to produce energy so that the excess fatty tissue around your body can be gradually broken down by the body for fuel. With time, this will lead to loss of weight and an improvement in your health.

Benefits of the Ketogenic Diet

So far we have discussed what the Ketogenic diet is and how it changes your body's metabolism. But what good does all this do from a health perspective? Let's look at some of the benefits of this diet in greater detail.

1. It breaks down the excess fatty tissue in your body for energy production, thus making you leaner and healthier.

2. Less insulin is produced in the body, thus allowing greater production of hormones that promote fat burning. This also helps in regulation of blood sugar levels.

3. Your body will no longer experience energy surges and drops as you would with a high-carb diet. This means that you will have greater and more stable energy levels as your body becomes more efficient in energy

production.

4. Studies show that a high-fat low-carb diet can help athletes improve their endurance. It minimizes oxidative stress, increases the mitochondrial levels, and reduces lactic acid during sports. This can be beneficial for you when exercising.

5. The aging process is slowed down, thus making you look much younger and vibrant. As the levels of oxidative stress are reduced, your lifespan is ultimately increased.

6. The functioning of your brain is boosted. You will begin to experience clearer thoughts, a higher learning capacity, and improvement in memory.

7. There is a reduction in inflammation and greater pain relief. The process of ketosis tends to strengthen your nervous system, thus raising your pain threshold. Consuming fewer carbohydrates translates to less glucose metabolism, which promotes anti-inflammation.

8. The Ketogenic diet helps to reverse certain cardiovascular and metabolic ailments.

9. The diet relieves the symptoms associated with Irritable Bowel Syndrome (IBS), such as stomach pain, diarrhea, and bloating.

These are just 9 of the major benefits that the Ketogenic diet will give you. The Ketogenic diet is suitable for anyone who wants to lose weight and improve their health. The important thing is to know your body and what you want to achieve.

Chapter 2:

Cleaning Out Your Pantry

Before you launch into your Ketogenic journey, it is important that you first consider planning your route. One of the first things you will have to do is clean out your kitchen pantry. This is important because you want to eliminate all kinds of temptation that may ruin your chances of achieving your weight loss goals.

So where or how do you even start? Follow this kitchen pantry guide.

Snacks

These are some of the snacks that you may have to toss out. Of course, you can easily replace them with some more keto-friendly items. For example:

- Replace potato chips with seaweed snacks, nuts, seeds, beef jerky, or veggie chips.

- Replace cookies with no-sugar biscuits.

- Replace chocolate with no-sugar chocolate sweetened with Stevia.

- Replace breakfast cereals with Atkins low-carb bars.

- Replace any low-fat snacks with the full-fat version.

Ingredients

There are some basic cooking and baking ingredients that are full of carbs and must be replaced. For example:

- Replace wheat flours with coconut or almond flour.

- Replace rice with chopped up cauliflower.

- Replace sugars with Stevia, Splenda, or Erythritol.

- Replace corn starch/flour with Xanthan gum.

- Buy low-carb pasta (Konjac noodles, Ciao proto pasta) instead of regular pasta.

- Remove any spreads with added sugar.

- Remove any sauces with a carb count of more than 10 grams per serving.

Ketogenic Grocery List

Now that you've cleared out the former junk, you have to fill that empty space with something much healthier. Here is a list of some ideal Ketogenic foods that you may want to stock your pantry with:

Dairy

- Butter

- Cheese

- Sour cream

- Cream cheese

Protein/Meats

- Steak

- Ham

- Pepperoni

- Chicken

- Salami

- Bacon

- Sausage

- Pork loin

- Eggs

Nuts and Seeds

- Walnuts

- Sesame

- Pecans

- Almonds

- Flax

Fruits and Veggies

- Avocado

- Broccoli

- Asparagus

- Cucumbers

- Bell peppers

- Mushrooms

Dressings

- Lemon juice

- Lime juice

- Mayo

- Mustard

- Soy Sauce

Chapter 3:

Ketogenic Breakfast Recipes

If you are on a Ketogenic diet because you want to lose weight, then a healthy, hearty, Keto breakfast is the perfect way to start your day. A Ketogenic breakfast will give you the morning nutritional boost you need, as well as support your adrenal function, which is very important for weight loss. Be prepared to enjoy 14 super delicious breakfast recipes that will keep you satiated and not leave any room for possible cravings!

Please note that the carbohydrate quantities are in *net* grams since this is what ultimately matters in a low-carb diet.

KETO BREAKFAST FRITTATA

Ingredients:

4 large organic eggs
2 oz. full-fat Brie Cheese
1 avocado
10 Kalamata olives
2 Tbsp organic butter
1 tsp Herbs de Provence
2 Tbsp MCT oil
½ tsp Sea salt

Instructions:

Take a large bowl and pour in the eggs, MCT oil, and Herbs de Provence. Remove the pits from the olives before tossing them into the bowl. Use a whisk to make a frothy mixture.

Cut the avocado, peel it, and then slice into thick slices.

Place a large skillet over high heat and melt the butter. Toss in the avocado slices and fry them until they turn slightly golden. Use a spatula to remove them.

Pour the egg mixture into the same skillet. Cut thin slices of the cheese and place them on the egg mixture.

Place a lid over the skillet and wait for 3 minutes for the frittata to turn golden brown.
Flip the frittata and cook the other side for 2 more minutes.
Serve hot with a topping of the fried avocado.

Nutritional information: 313 calories, 2.4 grams carbs, 9 grams protein, 30 grams fat.

CREAM CHEESE PANCAKES

Ingredients:

2 large pastured eggs
2 oz. cream cheese
1 tsp sugar substitute
½ tsp cinnamon

Instructions:

Take your blender and toss in all the ingredients, then blend until you get a smooth consistency.
Leave for 2 minutes for bubbles to settle.
Spray some butter on a pan and place over medium heat. Pour ¼ of the mixture into the pan.
Cook until golden brown before flipping onto the other side. Cook for an additional 1 minute.
Repeat the process using the mixture that is remaining.
Serve with fresh berries.

Nutritional information: 344 calories, 2.5 grams carbs, 17 grams protein, 29 grams fat.

KETO CEREAL WITH CACAO NIBS

Ingredients:

1 cup water
½ cup chia seeds
2 Tbsp raw cacao nibs
2 Tbsp melted coconut oil
4 Tbsp hemp hearts
1 Tbsp Swerve
1 Tbsp Psyllium powder
1 Tbsp vanilla extract

Instructions:

Preheat the oven to 285 degrees F.
Take a large mixing bowl, pour in the water and chia seeds, and leave for 5 minutes.
Break the cacao nibs into smaller chunks and then add all the ingredients into the bowl. Use a wooden spoon to mix all the ingredients together until it forms a ball of dough.
Spread out two pieces of parchment paper. Using your hands, mold the dough into a cylinder and then place it on one of the parchment papers. Make sure the shiny side of the paper is facing up.
Flatten the dough using your fingers and then cover it with the second parchment paper, shiny side down.

Use a rolling pin to roll the dough to a thickness of ¼ inch.

Remove the top parchment and place the dough on a cookie sheet. Put the dough into the oven for 15 minutes and then flip it. Bake the other side for another 15 minutes.

Remove from oven and cool.

Use a knife to slice the baked cereal into squares measuring 1 inch in length.

Serve in a bowl of milk.

Nutritional information per serving: 254 calories, 1.5 grams carbs, 9.2 grams protein, 15.5 grams fats

FRENCH TOAST WITH PUMPKIN SPICE

Ingredients:

4 slices pumpkin bread
2 Tbsp butter
2 Tbsp cream
1 large egg
½ tsp vanilla extract
1/8 tsp orange extract
¼ tsp Pumpkin Pie Spice

Instructions:

Keep the bread slices in the open to dry them out overnight.
Take a large mixing bowl and toss in the egg, extracts, cream, and pumpkin pie spice.
Place the slices of bread in the bowl to soak up the mixture. Make sure both sides of each slice soak up the mixture.
Place the butter in a pan over medium heat. When the butter turns brown, place the slices in the pan. When one side turns brown, flip over and do the other side.
Serve with Keto maple syrup.

Nutritional information per serving: 428 calories, 6.8 grams carbs, 12 grams protein, 37.4 grams fats.

MOCCA CHIA PUDDING

Ingredients:

1/3 cup coconut cream
1/3 cup chia seeds
2 cups water
1 Tbsp Swerve
2 Tbsp herbal coffee
2 Tbsp cacao nibs
1 Tbsp vanilla extract

Instructions:

Boil the water, add the herbal coffee, and allow to simmer for 15 minutes.
Sieve the herbal coffee and then add the swerve, extract, and coconut cream into the coffee pot. Add the cacao nibs and chia seeds into the pot and stir well.
Pour the mixture into serving bowls and put the containers in the fridge for 30 minutes.
Serve chilled.

Nutritional information per serving: 257 calories, 2.25 grams carbs, 7 grams protein, 21 grams fat.

ITALIAN BREAKFAST CASSEROLE

Ingredients:

4 large organic eggs
1 large spaghetti squash
A handful Italian parsley, chopped
3 oz. Italian salami, sliced
½ cup kalamata olives, halved
1 cup onion, diced
½ cup organic tomatoes, diced
2 cloves minced garlic
4 Tbsp bacon fat
½ tsp dried Italian seasoning
Black pepper and salt to taste

Instructions:

Preheat the oven to 400 degrees F.
Cut the squash into two halves and remove the seeds. Place the two halves facing up on a baking sheet.
Spread 2 Tbsp of the bacon fat over the top surface of each squash. Sprinkle the black pepper and salt over the bacon fat. Place in oven and bake for 45 minutes.
Place an oven-proof skillet over medium heat and add the remaining 2 Tbsp of bacon fat. Then toss in the onions and garlic. Add salt and pepper to taste.

When the mixture starts to thicken, toss in the tomatoes and slices of salami. Sauté for 10 minutes before adding the kalamata olives.

Remove the squash from the oven. Using a fork, scrape out the flesh from the two squash halves. Toss in the flesh into the skillet.

Take a large spoon and dig 4 deep holes in the mixture. Then crack the eggs, one over each hole.

Remove the skillet from the heat and place it in the oven. Bake until the egg whites are well done.

Top off with the chopped parsley.

Serve and enjoy!

Nutritional information per serving: 333 calories, 13.25 grams carbs, 14 grams protein, 23 grams fats.

BREAKFAST BURGER

Ingredients:

2 large eggs
4 slices bacon
4 oz. sausage
2 oz. Pepperjack cheese
1 Tbsp PB Fit powder
1 Tbsp butter
Salt and pepper to taste

Instructions:

Preheat the oven to 400 degrees F.
Bake the bacon slices in the oven for 25 minutes.
In a mixing bowl, whisk together the PB Fit powder and the butter. Set the bowl aside.
Use your hands to form sausage patties. Place a pan over medium heat and cook the sausages. Toss in the cheese and then cover the pan. Remove the sausages when they are well done.
Cook the eggs in the pan.
Assemble the bacon, sausage, and eggs.
Serve.

Nutritional information per serving: 655 calories, 3 grams carbs, 31 grams protein, 56 grams fats.

KETO LEMON POPPYSEED MUFFINS

Ingredients:

Zest of 2 lemons
3 large organic eggs
1/3 cup Erythritol
¼ cup melted salted butter
¼ cup heavy cream
¼ cup Golden Flaxseed Meal
¾ cup blanched almond flour
3 Tbsp lemon juice
2 Tbsp poppy seeds
1 tsp baking powder
25 drops Stevia
1 tsp vanilla extract

Instructions:

Preheat your oven to 350 degrees F.
In a small mixing bowl, pour in the almond flour, flax seed meal, erythritol, and poppy seeds.
Add the eggs, heavy cream, and melted butter into the bowl. Whisk until a smooth consistency is achieved.
Pour in the Stevia, vanilla extract, zest, lemon juice, and baking powder. Whisk thoroughly.
Pour the batter into 12 silicone cupcake molds. Alternatively, use a muffin pan.

Place the batter in the oven for 20 minutes. When ready, remove the mold and let the muffins cool for 10 minutes.
Slice the muffins and serve!

Nutritional information per muffin: 129 calories, 1.5 grams carbs, 3.7 grams protein, 11.5 grams fats.

WHITE CHEDDAR AND SAUSAGE BISCUITS

Ingredients:

1 large organic egg
1 cup white cheddar cheese, shredded
6 oz. sausage, cooked and thinly sliced
1 ½ cups almond flour
4 oz. cream cheese
¼ cup heavy cream
1/4 cup water
1 Tbsp chives, chopped
2 large cloves garlic, minced
½ tsp Italian seasoning
½ tsp sea salt

Instructions:

Preheat oven to 350 degrees F.
Take a medium bowl and pour in the eggs and cream cheese. Then use a hand mixer to whip the ingredients together.
Toss in the chives, garlic, Italian seasoning, and salt. Mix thoroughly.
Pour in the almond flour, heavy cream, cheddar cheese, and some water. Whip the mixture well.
Toss in the sausage pieces into the bowl and use a spatula to mix them in.

Take a muffin top pan, grease it lightly, and drop the batter into 8 of the wells.

Place the pan in the oven for 25 minutes. When ready, allow the pan to cool in the oven before removing.

Serve with a side of eggs and sliced tomatoes.

Nutritional information per serving: 321 calories, 3.5 grams, 13 grams protein, 28 grams fats.

KETO ZUCCHINI HASH

Ingredients:

1 medium-sized zucchini
1 large organic egg
2 slices bacon
1 Tbsp chives, chopped
1 Tbsp coconut oil
½ white onion
¼ tsp salt

Instructions:

Peel the onion and chop it finely. Slice the bacon into small pieces as well.

Place a pan over medium heat and pour in the coconut oil. Toss in the onions and then cook the bacon until light brown.

Chop the zucchini into medium pieces and toss them into the pan. Cook for 15 minutes.

Remove the pan from heat and place the food onto a serving plate. Top off with chopped chives and a fried egg. Add salt to taste.

Serve and enjoy!

Nutritional information per serving: 423 calories, 6.6 grams carbs, 7.4 grams protein, 36 grams fat

CREAM CHEDDAR WAFFLES

Ingredients:

3 oz. cream cheese
1 oz. Cheddar cheese
1 small Jalapeno
3 large organic eggs
1 tsp Psyllium Husk powder
1 Tbsp baking powder
1 Tbsp coconut flour
Salt and pepper

Instructions:

Place all the ingredients into a large mixing bowl and use an immersion blender to mix thoroughly. Heat the waffle pan and pour the mixture into it. When the waffles are ready, add your preferred topping.
Serve and enjoy!

Nutritional information per waffle: 340 calories, 3 grams carbs, 16 grams protein, 28 grams fat.

AVOCADO AND SALMON DELIGHT

Ingredients:

2 oz. wild salmon, smoked
1 oz. goat cheese
2 Tbsp extra virgin oil
1 organic avocado
Juice of 1 lemon
Sea salt to taste

Instructions:

Halve the avocado and remove the seed.
Put all the *other* ingredients in a food processor and
mix to achieve coarse consistency.
Pour the mixture into the avocado holes.
Serve!

Nutritional information per serving: 525 calories, 4
grams carbs, 19 grams protein, 48 grams fat.

CAJUN CAULI HASH

Ingredients:

8 oz. red pastrami, shaved
1 pound frozen cauliflower
1 large egg
½ green pepper
½ onion
2 Tbsp minced garlic
2 Tbsp ghee
1 tsp Cajun seasoning

Instructions:

Place a saucepan over medium heat, melt the ghee, and sauté the onions for 5 minutes.
Add the garlic and cook for 2 minutes.
Chop the cauliflower and steam it. Squeeze out the excess water, toss them into the pan, and sauté until crispy brown.
Add the Cajun seasoning, pastrami, and green peppers. Ensure all ingredients are well mixed.
When ready, put into serving bowls.
Fry the egg in the pan and use it as a topping. Add more seasoning if desired.

Nutritional information per serving: 486 calories, 7.3 grams carbs, 5.7 grams protein, 49 grams fat.

SWISS CHARD PIE

Ingredients:

8 cups Swiss chard
1 cup mozzarella, shredded
2 cups ricotta cheese
¼ cup parmesan, shredded
1 pound sausage
3 organic eggs
1 clove garlic, minced
½ cup onion, chopped
1 Tbsp olive oil
1/8 tsp ground nutmeg
Salt and pepper

Instructions:

Preheat the oven to 350 degrees F.
Take a large pan, pour in the olive oil, and sauté the onions and garlic. Cook until they turn soft.
Cook the Swiss chard in the pan for 5 minutes and then add the nutmeg, salt, and pepper. Remove the pan from heat.
Take a large bowl and beat the eggs, then add all the different cheeses. Pour the sautéed Swiss chard into the bowl and stir.

Press the sausage uniformly into a large pie tin.
Pour the filling into the pie tin, put it on a cookie
sheet, and place in the oven. Bake for half an hour
until the pie becomes firm.
Remove and allow to cool. Top off with more cheese
as desired.
Serve.

Nutritional information per serving: 344 calories, 4
grams carbs, 2 grams protein, 27 grams fat.

Chapter 4:

Ketogenic Lunch Recipes

For most working people, getting a healthy lunch in a restaurant can be quite challenging. This is especially true for those on a Ketogenic diet. In this chapter, you will learn 14 of the easiest Keto lunches that you can make at home and carry to work with you. Not only are these meals delicious, they will also save you time and help you stick to a healthier way of enjoying your lunch break!

Please note that the carbohydrate quantities are in *net* grams since this is what ultimately matters in a low-carb diet.

KETO-STUFFED AVOCADO

Ingredients:

1 large avocado
3.2 oz. sardines
0.5 oz. chives
1 Tbsp mayo
1 Tbsp lemon juice
¼ tsp ground turmeric root
¼ tsp salt

Instructions:

Cut the avocado in half and remove the seed.
Remove the sardines from the tin and drain them.
Put them in a bowl and use a fork to break them
into tiny pieces.
Use a spoon to scoop out the flesh from the center of
the avocado. Leave about ½ inch of flesh.
Finely chop the chives and grate the turmeric root.
Pour both into the bowl containing sardines. Add
the mayonnaise and mix well.
Toss the avocado flesh into the bowl and mash it as
desired. Add the lemon juice and season with salt.
Scoop the mixture into each avocado well.
Serve and enjoy!

Nutritional information per serving: 633 calories,
5.5 grams carbs, 27.2 grams protein, 52.6 grams fats.

BLACKBERRY CHIPOTLE CHICKEN WINGS

Ingredients:

½ cup Blackberry Chipotle Jam
3 pounds chicken wings
½ cup water
Salt and pepper to taste

Instructions:

Preheat the oven to 400 degrees F.
Chop up the wings by splitting the drummettes from the wing tips.
Take a medium mixing bowl and pour in the jam, then add water. Use a whisk to mix thoroughly.
Place the chicken wings into a plastic Ziploc bag and pour in 2/3 of the jam marinade. Add the salt and pepper and lock the bag. Leave for half an hour.
Place the marinated chicken wings on a cookie sheet and bake for 15 minutes. Flip the chicken pieces over and brush the remaining marinade over them.
Increase heat to 425 degrees F and bake for half an hour.
Serve hot!

Nutritional information per wing: 503 calories, 1.8 grams carbs, 34.5 grams protein, 40 grams fat.

LOW-CARB AVOCADO SUSHI

Ingredients:

1 avocado
2 oz. smoked salmon, sliced
18 oz. cauliflower, riced
1 Tbsp rice vinegar
2 Tbsp butter
4 Nori papers
Cream cheese, whipped

Instructions:

Place a pan over medium heat and melt the butter.
Add the cauliflower and sauté for 10 minutes.
As the cauliflower cools, take the nori papers and
use the cream cheese to coat them.
Stir the vinegar into the pan with cauliflower.
Place the cauliflower mixture in a thin layer onto the
cream cheese.
On the edges of the nori paper, place the avocado
and salmon slices.
Roll the paper and cut.
Serve!

Nutritional information per roll: 335 calories, 5.3
grams carbs, 11.5 grams protein, 28.5 grams fat.

ALMOND BUTTER AND BACON BURGER

Ingredients:

For Almond Butter Sauce:
1 cup water
1 cup almond butter
6 Tbsp coconut amino
1 Tbsp rice vinegar
1 tsp Swerve
4 chili peppers
4 cloves garlic, peeled

For the Burger:
8 slices bacon, uncured
4 slices Pepper Jack Cheese
1.5 pounds pastured ground beef
8 leaves Romaine lettuce
1 large red onion
Black pepper and sea salt to taste

Instructions:

For Sauce:
Pour the water and almond butter into a saucepan and mix well. Place the pan over low heat and stir until the mixture thickens.
Toss in the coconut aminos and stir.

As the mixture continues cooking, place the peppers, garlic, vinegar, and swerve into a small food processor. Blend to a smooth consistency. Pour the smooth paste into the saucepan and continue stirring until well mixed.

Set aside.

For Burger:

Take the ground beef and form 4 patties. Use your thumb to make an indentation in the center of the patties to prevent them from becoming round when cooked.

Put the patties in a broiler pan and sprinkle salt and pepper over them.

Heat up the oven and place the broiler pan in. Leave until the top of the patties turn golden brown, then remove the patties and flip them over. Put them back in the oven and broil them for another 7 minutes.

Remove the burgers and place slices of cheese on them. Then return them to the oven to melt the cheese.

In the meantime, fry the bacon in a skillet and then cut the onion into ¼" slices.

Assemble the burger by taking 4 serving plates and placing 2 lettuce leaves on each plate. Place the burgers on the lettuce, followed by the onion slices. Top off with the bacon slices and pour almond sauce.

Serve and enjoy!

Nutritional information per serving: 890 calories, 8 grams carbs, 54 grams protein, 68 grams fat.

KETO CAESAR SALAD

Ingredients:

4 anchovy filets
2 oz. pork rinds
1 egg yolk
24 leaves Romaine hearts
2 cloves garlic
8 Tbsp avocado oil
4 Tbsp Parmesan, shaved
3 Tbsp Apple Cider vinegar
4 Tbsp Parmesan, grated
1 tsp Dijon mustard

Instructions:

Pour the yolk, mustard, and vinegar into a bowl.
Insert an immersion blender into the bowl and hold
it in place over the egg yolk. As you pour the
avocado oil into the bowl, run the blender on low.
The yolk will emulsify together with the avocado oil
to form a mayonnaise.
Toss in the grated parmesan, garlic, and anchovies.
Blend the ingredients slowly to form a smooth
mayo mixture.
Clean the romaine leaves and dry them before
placing them on 4 serving plates.
Use a spoon to drizzle the mayo dressing over the
leaves.

Chop the pork rinds into small pieces and share between the plates.
Use the shaved parmesan as a garnish.

Nutritional instructions per serving: 727 calories, 1.8 grams carbs, 13 grams protein, 38.75 grams fat.

THAI COCONUT SOUP WITH SHRIMP

Ingredients:

For the Broth:
1 ½ cups coconut milk
4 cups chicken broth
1 cup fresh cilantro
Zest of 1 organic lime
1 tsp dried lemongrass
1 tsp sea salt
1" fresh ginger root
1 jalapeno, sliced

For the Soup:
3.5 oz. raw wild shrimp
1 oz. mushrooms, sliced
1 oz. red onion, thinly sliced
1 Tbsp fish sauce
1 Tbsp cilantro, chopped
1 Tbsp coconut oil
Juice of 1 lime

Instructions:

Place a saucepan over low heat and put all the ingredients for the broth into it. Simmer lightly for 20 minutes.
Pour the broth through a strainer and collect the liquid. Pour the liquid back into the saucepan.

As the broth continues simmering, add the shrimp and fish sauce.

Toss in the coconut oil, mushrooms, and sliced onions. Allow simmering for 10 minutes until the shrimp is cooked.

Pour in the lime juice.

Place in 2 serving bowls and garnish with chopped cilantro.

Nutritional information per serving: 493 calories, 8 grams carbs, 11.5 grams protein, 45.3 grams fat

PUMPKIN CARBONARA

Ingredients:

1 packet Shiritaki noodles
2 pastured eggs
5 oz. Pancetta
1/3 cup parmesan
¼ cup heavy cream
3 Tbsp pumpkin puree
2 Tbsp butter
½ tsp dried sage
Salt and pepper to taste

Instructions:

Place the noodles in a bowl of hot water for 3 minutes, and then dry them out.

Cut the Pancetta, heat up a pan, and place it into the hot pan until it becomes crisp. Remove the Pancetta and keep the leftover fat for later use.

Take a pot, place over medium heat, and melt the butter until it turns brown.

Add the sage and pumpkin puree, and then toss in the leftover Pancetta fat and heavy cream. Mix well.

Put the noodles in the pan that cooked the Pancetta and heat on High. Fry until they dry out.

Add the parmesan into the pot containing pumpkin sauce and mix. Lower heat and stir to thicken the sauce.

Pour the noodles and Pancetta into the sauce and mix well. Finally, pour in the egg yolks and stir well.
Serve.

Nutritional information per serving: 384 calories, 2 grams carbs, 14 grams protein, 35 grams fat.

KETO LIVER PATE

Ingredient:

3 oz. leftover chicken liver, sautéed
3 tbsp organic butter
1 tsp chopped thyme
1 tsp chopped sage
1 tsp chopped oregano
Sea salt and ground black pepper to taste

Instructions:

Place every ingredient into a food processor. Mix to form a smooth paste.
Serve with raw crackers or slices of radish.

Nutritional information per serving: 381 calories, 1 gram carbs, 17 grams protein, 40 grams fat.

MEAT MUFFINS

Ingredients:

1 pound organic ground beef
½ pound mushrooms
6 organic eggs
¾ cup organic coconut flour
2 Tbsp coconut aminos
1 tsp sea salt

Instructions:

Preheat the oven to 350 degrees F.
Place the mushrooms in a large food processor and chop them up. Toss in the eggs, aminos, and salt. Mix all the ingredients to form a smooth puree. Pour out the egg and mushroom mixture into a large mixing bowl. Mix in the ground beef and coconut flour. Make sure the flour has been sifted. The dough formed should be soft yet firm enough to form meatballs.
Lay out 13 cupcake cups on a cookie sheet. Mold the dough into balls and place into each cup.
Bake the cupcakes for 45 minutes until the meatballs turn brown on top.
Serve warm or cold.

Nutritional information per serving: 165 calories, 1 gram carbs, 12 grams protein, 10 grams fat.

FRESH KETO CHILI

Ingredients:

2 pounds ground beef
8 cups spinach
1 cup tomato sauce
2 green peppers
1 small onion
1 Tbsp chili powder
1 Tbsp curry powder
1 Tbsp olive oil
1 Tbsp cumin
1 tsp Xanthan gum
1 tsp garlic powder
2 tsp cayenne pepper

Instructions:

Place the beef in a pot and cook until it turns brown.
Add all the spices and mix well.
Chop the onions and bell peppers, and sauté them
using olive oil in a separate pan. Use medium heat.
Add the spinach into the pan with beef. Stir and
cook. Add the tomato sauce, mix, and cook for 10
minutes.
Pour the onions and peppers into the beef mixture
and stir. Add 1 tsp of the Xanthan gum and mix
thoroughly until the stew thickens.
Serve hot topped with cheese.

Nutritional information per serving: 357 calories, 4.5 grams carbs, 31 grams protein, 22 grams fat.

KETO PIZZA

Ingredients:

For the crust:
1 cup water
1 cup chia seeds
3 Tbsp olive oil
1 medium cauliflower
1 tsp sea salt

For Topping:
2 cloves garlic
½ cup cream cheese
½ cup heavy cream
½ cup grated parmesan

Instructions:

Preheat the oven to 100 degrees F.
Chop off the florets from the cauliflower and toss them into a food processor.
Use a coffee grinder to grind the chia seeds.
Take a large mixing bowl and pour in the cauliflower, chia flour, olive oil, water, and salt. Mix thoroughly to form a smooth dough. Set aside for 20 minutes.
Meanwhile, lightly spread some olive oil on a cookie sheet.

Spread the dough mixture about ½" thick over the cookie sheet.

Bake for an hour until the crust becomes dry. Once crust dries, increase the temperature of the oven to 400 degrees F.

To make the Keto topping, place the cream, cheese, and garlic in a food processor. Mix to form a smooth paste. Spread this paste over the pizza crust and bake for another 10 minutes.

Serve.

Nutritional information per serving: 398 calories, 3 grams carbs, 13.5 grams protein, 30 grams fat.

SUNDAY LUNCHROAST

Ingredients:

5 pounds beef rib roast
1 tsp salt
1 tsp garlic powder
1 tsp pepper

Instructions:

Preheat the oven to 375 degrees F.
Leave the beef roast to stand for 1 hour at room temperature.
Mix all the spices together; place the roast on the roasting rack and spread the spices over the meat.
Place the roast in the oven for 1 hour, and then switch off the oven.
Leave the roast to cool for about 15 minutes.
Cut and serve.

Nutritional information per serving: 681 calories, 0.3 grams, carbs, 90 grams protein, 50 grams fat.

PESTO EGG MUFFINS

Ingredients:

6 large organic eggs
2/3 cup fresh spinach
¼ cup chopped tomatoes
½ cup kalamata
4.4 oz. goat cheese
3 Tbsp pesto
Salt and pepper to taste

Instructions:

Preheat the oven to 350 degrees F.
Blanch the spinach in boiling water for 1 minute and
then dip in cold water to stop it cooking. Squeeze
out the water.
Remove the seeds from the olives and slice the
tomatoes.
Take a mixing bowl and pour in the egg yolks. Add
the pesto, salt, and pepper. Mix thoroughly.
Take the silicon muffin pan and split the spinach,
tomatoes, cheese, and olives uniformly between the
wells of the pan. Pour in the egg-pesto mixture and
place the pan in the oven.
Bake for 25 minutes until cooked through.
Remove from oven and allow to cool.
Enjoy!

Nutritional information per serving: 125 calories, 1.2 grams carbs, 6.9 grams protein, 10.2 grams fat.

LONDON BROIL

Ingredients:

2 pounds London Broil
½ cup coffee
¼ cup white wine
½ cup chicken broth
1 Tbsp soy sauce
1 Tbsp Dijon mustard
2 Tbsp reduced sugar ketchup
2 tsp onion powder
2 tsp garlic, minced

Instructions:

Place the London Broil in a slow cooker.
In a mixing bowl, add the soy sauce, Dijon, ketchup, and garlic. Mix well to form a marinade.
Spread the marinade over the sides of the Broil and sprinkle the onion powder over the top.
Pour all the liquid ingredients into the slow cooker.
Set the temperature on High.
Cook for 5 hours and then use a fork to rip the meat.
Serve and enjoy.

Nutritional information per serving: 410 calories, 2.5 grams carbs, 47 grams protein, 19 grams fat.

Chapter 5:

Ketogenic Dinner Delights

Most people who live a Ketogenic lifestyle are always on the lookout for great keto dinner recipes that are quick and easy to make. This chapter offers you 14 fabulous dinner recipes packed with everything you need to stay keto! Enjoy!

Please note that the carbohydrate quantities are in *net* grams since this is what ultimately matters in a low-carb diet.

BUTTERED EGGS

Ingredients:

4 pastured eggs
2 cloves garlic, chopped
½ cup parsley, chopped
½ cup cilantro, chopped
1 Tbsp coconut oil
2 Tbsp pastured butter
1 tsp fresh thyme
¼ tsp ground cayenne
¼ tsp ground cumin
½ tsp sea salt

Instructions:

Place a non-stick skillet over a low flame to heat the butter and coconut oil for 1 minute.
Cook the garlic for 3 minutes until it turns brown.
Add the thyme and cook for another 30 seconds.
Increase to medium heat and then add the parsley and cilantro. Cook until the herbs turn crisp.
Crack the eggs directly into the skillet, cover it, and reduce to low heat. Cook for 5 minutes.
Serve immediately with sausages.

Nutritional information per serving: 311 calories, 2.5 grams carbs, 13 grams protein, 28 grams fat.

WEEKEND BEEF ROAST

Ingredients:

5 pounds beef rib roast
1 tsp pepper
1 tsp garlic powder
2 tsp salt

Instructions:

Preheat the oven to 375 degrees F.
Let the roast stand for an hour to attain room temperature.
In a small mixing bowl, mix the salt, pepper, and garlic.
Put the roast ribs on a roasting rack and smear the spices over the beef.
Place the beef ribs in the oven for an hour and then switch off the oven. Keep the door closed and let the roast stay there for 3 hours.
Turn the oven back on and warm the roast for 30 minutes at 375 degrees F.
Remove the roast and cool it for 10 minutes.
Cut and serve.

Nutritional information per serving: 681 calories, 0.4 grams carbs, 90 grams protein, 46.6 grams fat.

TUNA AND AVOCADO BALLS

Ingredients:

10 oz. canned tuna, drained
1 large avocado, cubed
¼ cup mayonnaise
1/3 cup almond flour
½ cup coconut oil
¼ cup parmesan cheese
¼ tsp onion powder
½ tsp garlic powder
Salt and pepper to taste

Instructions:

Take a large mixing bowl and put in all the
ingredients, except the avocado, almond flour, and
coconut oil. Mix thoroughly.
Cut the avocado into cubes and add to the tuna mix.
Make some tuna balls and pour the flour over them.
Place a pan over medium heat and add coconut oil.
Fry the tuna balls until all sides are brown.
Serve.

Nutritional information per ball: 135 calories, 0.8
grams carbs, .2 grams protein, 11.8 grams fat.

PORK SMOKIE WRAPS

Ingredients:

37 Lit'l Smokies
1 large egg
1 ½ oz. cream cheese
8 oz. cheddar cheese
¾ cup almond flour
1 Tbsp Psyllium Husk powder
1/2 tsp pepper
½ tsp salt

Instructions:

Preheat the oven to 400 degrees F.
Place the cheddar cheese in the microwave. Heat the cheese at 20-second intervals until it starts bubbling.
In a mixing bowl, combine all the ingredients, including the melted cheddar cheese, to form dough.
Lay the dough on parchment paper and then place it in the fridge for 20 minutes to harden.
Remove the dough, lay it on foil, and slice it into strips. Use the dough strips to wrap the Lit'l Smokies.
Bake in the oven for 15 minutes and then broil for another 2 minutes.
Serve warm!

Nutritional instructions per Smokie: 72 calories, 0.6 grams carbs, 3.9 grams protein, 6 grams fat.

MIXED GREEN SPRING SALAD

Ingredients:

2 slices bacon
2 oz. Mixed Greens
2 Tbsp parmesan cheese, shaved
2 Tbsp Keto Raspberry Vinaigrette
3 Tbsp roasted pine nuts
Salt and pepper

Instructions:

Fry the bacon in a pan until it becomes crispy.
In a large mixing bowl, place all the other
ingredients. Crumble the bacon into the bowl.
Mix the salad well and serve.

Nutritional information per serving: 478 calories,
4.4 grams carbs, 17 grams protein, 37 grams fat.

CHICKEN AND ZUCCHINI

Ingredients:

6 oz. Rotisserie chicken
3 oz. cheddar cheese
10 oz. zucchini
1 stalk green onion
1 cup broccoli, chopped
2 Tbsp sour cream
2 Tbsp butter, melted
Salt and pepper to taste

Instructions:

Preheat the oven to 400 degrees F.
Halve the zucchini lengthwise.
Using a spoon, scoop out the flesh until you remain with the zucchini shell.
Pour the butter into the shell and add salt and pepper.
Bake in the oven for 20 minutes.
Shred the chicken.
Place the chopped broccoli into a bowl and then add the sour cream, salt, and pepper.
When the zucchini is ready, remove from the oven and place the chicken and broccoli into the shells.
Sprinkle the cheddar cheese over the filling and bake in the oven for 15 more minutes.
Top off using green onions and sour cream.

Serve.

Nutritional information per zucchini shell: 530 calories, 5 grams carbs, 30 grams protein, 35 grams fat.

SPICED PUMPKIN SOUP

Ingredients:

4 slices bacon
1 Bay leaf
2 cloves roasted garlic, minced
¼ medium onion, chopped
1 cup Pumpkin Puree
1.5 cups chicken broth
½ cup heavy cream
4 Tbsp butter
3 Tbsp bacon grease
1/8 tsp nutmeg
½ tsp fresh ginger, minced
¼ tsp cinnamon
½ tsp pepper
¼ tsp coriander
½ tsp salt

Instructions:

Place a saucepan over medium heat and brown the butter. Add the onions, garlic, and ginger, and cook for 2 minutes.

When the onions turn translucent, add spices and stir. Wait for 2 minutes before adding the chicken broth and pumpkin puree. Stir thoroughly.

Bring mixture to a boil and then reduce heat.
Simmer for 20 minutes and then dip an immersion
blender into the pan to blend until smooth.
Let the soup simmer for an extra 20 minutes as you
cook the bacon slices.
When the soup is ready, pour in the bacon grease
and heavy cream. Stir the soup thoroughly.
Crumble the bacon and sprinkle it over the soup.
Serve.

Nutritional information per serving: 485 calories, 7
grams carbs, 6 grams protein, 49 grams fat.

KETO PORK SOUP

Ingredients:

1 pound pork shoulder, sliced and cooked
2 cups bone broth
2 cups chicken broth
6 oz. mushrooms
½ green pepper, sliced
½ red Bell pepper, sliced
½ jalapeno, sliced
½ medium onion
¼ cup tomato paste
½ cup strong coffee
2 Bay leaves
Juice of ½ lime
2 tsp chili powder
2 tsp cumin
½ tsp pepper
¼ tsp cinnamon
1 tsp oregano
1 tsp paprika
1 tsp garlic, minced
½ tsp salt

Instructions:

Place a saucepan over high heat and add the olive oil. Chop the onions and sauté. Remove the pan from heat before the onions turn brown.

Place the pork slices in a slow cooker and add the mushrooms, broths, and coffee.
Add spices and the rest of the herbs. Stir well and cover with a lid. Cook for 5 hours.
Serve.

Nutritional information per serving: 386 calories, 6.4 grams carbs, 20 grams protein, 30 grams fat.

KETO PESTO CHICKEN SALAD

Ingredients:

1 pound chicken, cooked and cubed
6 slices bacon, cooked and crumbled
10 tomatoes, halved
1 avocado, cubed
¼ cup mayonnaise
2 Tbsp garlic pesto

Instructions:

Take a large mixing bowl and put in the tomatoes, chicken, bacon, avocado, and pesto. Toss the ingredients gently to ensure even coating.

Nutritional information per serving: Calories 375, 3 grams carbs, 27 grams protein, 30 grams fat.

SPICY CHICKEN SATAY

Ingredients:

1 pound chicken, ground
2 spring onions
1 yellow pepper
Juice of ½ lime
4 Tbsp soy sauce
3 Tbsp peanut butter
1 Tbsp rice vinegar
1 Tbsp Erythritol
¼ tsp paprika
1 tsp garlic, minced
2 tsp chili paste
2 tsp sesame oil
¼ tsp cayenne

Instructions:

Place a skillet over medium heat and pour in the sesame oil.
Cook the ground chicken until it turns brown and then toss in all the other ingredients, except the onions and yellow pepper. Stir well and cook the meat all the way through.
Add the onions and yellow pepper.
Serve and enjoy!

Nutritional information per serving: 395 calories, 3.8 grams carbs, 33 grams protein, 24 grams fat.

KETO SWEDISH MEATBALLS

Ingredients:

1 large pastured egg
2 pounds ground meat (1 pound beef and pork)
15 cups heavy cream
15 cups chicken broth
1 cup cheddar cheese, shredded
¼ cup diced onions
1 Tbsp Worcestershire sauce
1 Tbsp Dijon mustard
4 Tbsp salted butter
4 Tbsp water
¼ tsp allspice
½ tsp ground nutmeg

Instructions:

Preheat the oven to 400 degrees F.
Preheat slow cooker on Low setting.
Place the ground meat in a large bowl together with the egg, cheese, onion, allspice, nutmeg, and water. Mix and roll into 1 ½ inch balls.
Take a large baking pan and line it with parchment paper. Place the meatballs on the pan. You can use two baking pans if necessary.
Place the baking pan in the oven for 20 minutes.

Place a skillet over medium heat and melt the butter. Pour in the chicken broth and heavy cream and cook until mixture simmers. Lower heat and allow to simmer for another 20 minutes. Stir regularly.

Add the Worcestershire sauce and mustard. Stir well and then pour the sauce into the slow cooker. Remove the meatballs from the oven and toss them into the sauce.

Cook for 2 hours on low heat setting. Stir every 30 minutes.

Serve.

Nutritional information per meatball: 773 calories, 3 grams carbs, 74 grams protein, 50 grams fat.

KOREAN BARBEQUE BOWL

Ingredients:

1 pound skirt steak, thinly sliced
2 cloves garlic
2 cups riced cauliflower
4 Tbsp Sriracha sauce
2 Tbsp coconut oil
4 Tbsp coconut aminos
1 tsp ginger powder

Instructions:

In a mixing bowl, combine the sriracha, ginger, garlic, and coconut aminos to form a marinade.
Put the steak slices in a large Ziploc bag and pour in the marinade. Mix well.
Place in the fridge for 1 hour and remove 30 minutes prior to cooking.
Heat the coconut oil in a pan over high heat and add the cauliflower. Saute for 10 minutes as you stir regularly.
Place a 10 x 10 inch cast iron grill over high heat and grill the meat one slice at a time grill both sides until they are well done.
Pour the cauli rice in a serving bowl and add the steak slices on top.
Serve with chopped parsley.

Nutritional information per serving: 190 calories, 3.3 grams carbs, 16 grams protein, 10 grams fat.

KETO FISH FRITTERS

Ingredients:

4 eggs
6 oz. sardines
½ tsp salt
½ cup coconut flour
½ cup psyllium
2 cups cilantro

Instructions:

Place the sardines in a medium bowl and mash them into tiny pieces using a fork.

Add salt, eggs, and psyllium, and mix well. Leave for 5 minutes.

Finely chop the cilantro and toss into the bowl. Mix well to form a spongy dough mixture.

Make 12 patties from the dough, each about 2 inches wide and ¾ inch thick. Dredge the patties in coconut flour.

Place a non-stick skillet over medium heat and pour in 1 Tbsp of the coconut oil. Fry the patties in batches of 3, with each batch consuming 1 Tbsp of oil.

Fry each patty for 3 minutes per side. Clean the pan between each batch of patties to remove traces of flour.

Place the patties on absorbent paper.

Serve 3 patties per person.

Nutritional information per portion: 269 calories, 1.8 grams carbs, 16 grams protein, 23 grams fat.

FRIED COD WITH AVOCADO CREAM

Ingredients:

For Fish:
1 pound fresh cod
2 egg whites
3 Tbsp coconut oil
½ cup coconut flour
½ tsp sea salt

For Dressing:
½ cup coconut cream
1/3 serrano pepper
1 medium avocado
½ Tbsp cilantro, chopped
½ tsp ginger, grated
1 tsp sea salt
1 tsp fresh lemon juice

Instructions:

Take a small bowl and whisk together the egg whites and salt.
Sieve the flour into a large plate.
Chop the cod into 4 fillets, dip them into the egg mixture, and finally dip them into the coconut flour. Coat evenly.
Place a large skillet over high heat and pour in the coconut oil.

Place the fillets into the hot oil gently. Cook for 2 minutes per side.

Reduce to medium flame and cook fillets for an extra 3 minutes until the fish flakes easily. Remove and lay on serving plates.

Take all the ingredients for the dressing and put into a food processor. Blend to form a smooth cream.

Dress the fillets in the cream.

Serve with salad.

Nutritional information per serving: 255 calories, 2 grams carbs, 23 grams protein, 25 grams fat.

Chapter 6:

Ketogenic Dessert Treats

Looking for some delectable Ketogenic dessert recipes? Well, you have come to the right place! In this chapter, you will discover some of the tastiest low-carb no-sugar treats found anywhere. There are 7 dessert recipes here that are simply keto-indulgent and easy to make! Use them as part of your 14-day Ketogenic meal plan. Enjoy!

Please note that the carbohydrate quantities are in *net* grams since this is what ultimately matters in a low-carb diet.

KETO CHOCOLATE SOUFFLE

Ingredients:

6 large organic egg whites
3 large organic egg yolks
5 oz. unsweetened chocolate
1/3 cup Lakanto Monk Fruit sugar
1 Tbsp butter

Instructions:

Preheat the oven to 375 degrees F.
Smear butter on the insides of a soufflé dish.
Place a metallic bowl in a pan of simmering water
and pour the chocolate into the bowl. Stir until it
fully melts.
Remove the metal bowl from the pan, toss in the
yolks, and mix using a fork until it hardens.
Add the egg whites and a pinch of salt. Use an
electric mixer to blend at high speed. Slowly pour in
the Lakanto as you keep mixing.
Use a spatula to fold the mixture gently.
Pour the mixture into the soufflé dish and place in
the oven for 20 minutes. The top should be crusty
and the middle still jiggly.
Serve immediately.

Nutritional information per serving: 3.4 grams
carbs, 11 grams protein, 25 grams fat.

KETO BUTTERED CHOCOLATE

Ingredients:

4 oz. melted cacao butter
2 Tbsp Erythritol
2 oz. almond butter
2½ oz. sesame butter
½ tsp vanilla extract
A pinch of salt

Instructions:

Take a blender and pour in the sesame butter, almond butter, erythritol, salt and vanilla extract in that order.
Blend on low speed for 10 seconds, and then slowly pour in the cacao butter as you blend.
Blend fast for 15 seconds and then quickly pour into silicone molds.
Allow cooling for 1 hour before placing in the fridge.
Serve cold.

Nutritional information per serving: 146 calories, 1.5 grams, 2 grams protein, 15 grams fat.

CHIA AND COCONUT SQUARES

Ingredients:

1 cup coconut meat, dried and shredded
4 Tbsp chia seeds
½ cup cashews
½ cup water
1 Tbsp Swerve
1 Tbsp coconut oil
¼ tsp vanilla extract

Instructions:

Pour the water and chia seeds in a bowl and leave for 15 minutes.
Preheat the oven to 350 degrees F.
In a large mixing bowl, combine the soaked chia seeds, coconut oil shredded coconut, vanilla extract, and Swerve. Blend them well using your hands, and then toss in the cashews. Mix thoroughly.
Use parchment to line a 9 x 9-inch baking pan.
Place the mixture on the parchment paper and compress using your hands to be about ¾ inch thick. Bake until golden brown and dry in the center, which is about 45 minutes.
Allow to cool and then cut into 9 squares.

Nutritional information per serving: 164 calories, 3.5 grams carbs, 4 grams protein, 14 grams fat.

LEMON CURD

Ingredients:

12 Tbsp organic butter, melted
8 egg yolks
2 Tbsp vanilla extract
1/3 cup Swerve
½ cup fresh lemon juice
Zest of lemons used

Instructions:

Take a mixing bowl and add the zest, juice, yolks, Swerve, and vanilla. Whisk thoroughly until smooth mixture.
Toss in the melted butter and whisk well.
Place a pan over low flame and pour in the egg mixture. Stir often and cook for 10 minutes till the curd thickens.
Transfer the curd to a mason jar and refrigerate. Serve chilled.

Nutritional information per serving: 210 calories, 1.8 grams carbs, 3 grams protein, 21 grams fat.

COCO CHIA PUDDING

Ingredients:

1/3 cup chia seeds
2 Tbsp cacao nibs
1 tbsp swerve
2 Tbsp herbal coffee
1 tbsp vanilla extract
1/3 cup coconut cream

Instructions:

Take 2 cups of water and heat over low flame. Add the herbal coffee and simmer for 15 minutes.
Pour the coffee through a sieve and then add the coconut cream, Swerve, and vanilla extract.
Add chia seeds and the cacao nibs. Stir well.
Pour into 2 serving glasses and refrigerate for half an hour.
Serve.

Nutritional information per serving: 257 calories, 2.5 grams carbs, 7 grams protein, 20.5 grams fat.

KETO LIME PIE

Ingredients:

For the Crust:
1 egg
2 cups hazelnuts
1 Tbsp Swerve
1 Tbsp coconut oil
4 Tbsp organic butter, melted
4 Tbsp chia seeds

For Filling:
3 large eggs
½ cup sour cream
½ cup coconut cream
½ cup coconut shavings
1 cup key lime juice
1 Tbsp Key Lime zest
3 Tbsp Swerve

Instructions:

Preheat the oven to 375 degrees F.
Grind the hazelnuts into flour using a food processor. Add the eggs, Swerve, chia seeds, and butter. Blend the ingredients until dough is formed. Use the coconut oil to grease a 6 x 9-inch baking pan. Compress the dough flat onto the pan.
Bake for 20 minutes.

Meanwhile, prepare the filling by putting all filling ingredients into a large bowl. Use an immersion blender to mix until a smooth consistency is achieved.

Take the crust out of the oven, pour the filling over it, and put it back into the oven. Bake for another 45 minutes.

Take it out of the oven and set it aside to cool. Sprinkle the coconut flakes all over it and place in the fridge overnight.

Serve.

Nutritional information per portion: 466 calories, 7 grams carbs, 11 grams protein, 42 grams fat.

KETO MACAROON BITES

Ingredients:

3 egg whites
½ cup shredded coconut
¼ cup almond flour
1 Tbsp coconut oil
1 Tbsp vanilla extract
2 Tbsp Swerve

Instructions:

Preheat the oven to 400 degrees F.

Take a medium mixing bowl and pour in the almond flour, Swerve, and coconut shreds. Blend thoroughly.

In a small pan, heat the coconut oil and add the extract.

Meanwhile, place an empty bowl in the fridge.

Pour the melted coconut oil into the flour and mix well.

Remove the bowl from the fridge and toss in the egg whites. Whisk until the eggs become stiff.

Pour the whites into the flour and mix slowly to keep the eggs puffy.

Lay out 10 muffin cups and fill with the dough using a spoon.

Bake for 8 minutes until the macaroons turn slightly brown.

Take them out of the oven and allow to cool.
Serve.

Nutritional information per macaroon: 46 calories,
0.5 grams carbs, 1.8 grams protein, 5 grams fat.

Chapter 7:

Maintaining the Right Attitude

Everyone who has ever made any kind of meaningful change to their life has started by choosing their attitude and mindset. The same principle applies to anyone who wants to lose weight and improve their health. The battle may be to change the way your body looks and functions, but your attitude will definitely play a huge role as well. If you have the right mindset, you will find it much simpler to successfully implement the Ketogenic diet into your lifestyle and achieve your goals.

The first step in battling weight and health issues is to make up your mind that you are going to stick to the diet. The Ketogenic diet is not easy, especially the first few weeks when your body struggles to adapt to ketosis. Unfortunately, most people tend to give up during this period. Maybe it's because they didn't condition their minds from the beginning that they were going to persevere. It's easy to assume that your body will be your biggest enemy, but experience shows something much different. The battlefield is in your mind, and if you are serious about cutting down that fat, you will have to prepare yourself.

How to Develop Inner Motivation

You can achieve your weight loss and health goals; you just need to know how to recondition your mind to go about it. So what practical steps can you take to change your mental attitude and achieve these goals? How can you develop that inner motivation to keep you going? Follow these 7 key steps:

1. Wake up early in the morning and calculate your Body Mass Index (BMI). Measure your height and weight and use the BMI formula to determine how overweight you actually are. It is important to establish a baseline so that you start your Ketogenic diet with the information you need to lose weight healthily.

2. Sit down with pen and notepad and ask yourself why you want to lose weight. Note down briefly the major reasons why you feel it is important to lose weight and achieve good health. This is crucial because there will be times when you want to give up, but taking a good look at the list will help spur you on. Visualize the kind of life you will be living once you attain your weight loss goals. Create a personal connection with the reasons you list down.

3. On the same notepad, write down how being overweight has reduced the quality of your life. List down the ways that it damages your health and the potential diseases you will have to deal with if you don't take action.

4. Get your close relatives and friends to support you on your weight loss journey. Their help will come in handy when you start faltering, which is something you will have to watch out for. They can encourage you and even join you when exercising.

5. Once you have identified your weight loss goals and written them down, develop a practical plan. Go ahead and break the plan down into more manageable objectives. For example, losing 100 pounds isn't easy. However, if you focus on losing just 10 pounds every month, you will find the process much easier. You can also break down whatever other goals you have to fit your weekly or daily schedule.

6. Be clear about the type of meals you will be having and the exercise routines you will perform. Clarity is power, so write all this information down. Use the recipes provided in this book to help you launch your Ketogenic journey.

Specify the location, activities, time, and duration of the workouts you will be having.

7. Finally, learn to celebrate every small successful step you make. Don't be afraid to reward yourself whenever you achieve one of your goals and milestones. Of course, don't overdo it by consuming too much of a sugary treat that might have consequences later, but enjoy your successes along the way.

Ketogenic Success Tips for Beginners

There is no doubt that a Ketogenic diet will help you lose weight and improve your health. However, there are always some traps to watch out for. Please make sure that you always consult a doctor before engaging in any kind of diet.

Here are 4 tips to help you succeed:

1. Be prepared for a few weeks of fatigue and discomfort. The initial adaptation period usually takes a couple of weeks as your body transitions from burning glucose to fat. The good news is that once your body has adapted, you will feel more energetic than ever before since you won't be dealing with sugar spikes and dips.

2. It is likely that you will suffer from some micro-nutritional deficiencies due to lack of carbohydrates. However, you can mitigate against this by consuming enough fruits and vegetables. You should also consider taking Ketogenic supplements such as Omega-3, Taurine, Whey Protein, Spirulina, and others.

3. Avoid the Ketogenic diet if you happen to be diabetic in any way. This is because a diabetic cannot regulate the production of ketones in their bloodstream, which may lead to its overproduction. This may cause ketoacidosis, a very severe condition. This is why you are advised to consult your doctor first before going on a diet.

4. Resist the temptation to cheat by planning ahead. This diet may be easier to stick to at home, but when dealing with social events or eating out, things may get a bit tricky. If you are going to a restaurant, check its website for Ketogenic meals that you can order. If possible, you can also inquire about the types of foods that will be available at the social event you are attending.

The 7 steps outlined above and the 4 tips given here will help you get started on your Ketogenic weight loss journey. Maintaining the right attitude is critical for achieving your health goals, but you also have to plan ahead. Keep the tips given above in mind and you will enjoy your Ketogenic journey.

Chapter 8:

Intermittent Fasting

Now that you have read some delicious keto recipes we can talk about intermittent fasting. Intermittent fasting isn't a diet. It is more of a meal timing plan, where you focus on a period where you can eat any food you want and then you abstain from food for a longer period. In other words, you will not consume any calories for a set time interval. There will be a specific time where you can eat but that will be much shorter than the time you will be spending not eating.

Why would anyone do this?

This type of fasting is very powerful because of its health benefits. This is not a normal type of "diet" lifestyle and it will affect your everyday tasks. You should only do this for a couple of months and then take a break. The reason this type of fasting is worth talking about is because of the physical, cellular, and mental benefits.

What are the physical benefits?

This type of fasting causes dramatic fat loss. You could possibly lose about 10 pounds of complete fat in the first week. The best thing about losing fat so fast is that you preserve most of the muscle. Some diets make you lose weight fast but you are not just losing the fat, you are losing hard earned muscle as well. Another benefit is the increase in muscle density and muscle tone. Once the fat is being stripped away the muscle density goes up and your muscles look more toned. Another benefit is the improvement of vascular function making you look healthier and more attractive. It does this by improving skin completion and strengthening hair because of the nutrition uptake that occurs in the cells.

What are the physiological benefits?

Most people will start intermittent fasting because of the molecular and cellular benefits. Catecholamine's are hormones produced by the adrenal glands, which sit on top of the kidneys. The main catecholamine's are dopamine, epinephrine, and norepinephrine. Our friend epinephrine will do something very special to us when we start to fast. Once we go into an extended period of time without eating, epinephrine will use fat reserves as metabolic energy and preserve muscle. Many hormones will help you preserve muscle but epinephrine is just one of them.

What are the mental benefits?

 When you are intermittent fasting, your brain goes into survival mode. This causes you to become hyper focused. The brain wants you to preserve energy for the task at hand. This will help you find true focus. An example of you feeling this type of hyper focus is when you have to wake up early for some important reason. Let's say you wake up at 5am to study for an exam at 9am. You went to bed at 8pm and all you can think about when you wake up at 5am is the test at 9am. During those 4 hours where you want to study as much as you can, you are hyper focused at the task at hand which is studying. You didn't care about eating or anything else. What you just did was enter in an extended period of not eating, which caused hormones to use fat storage as energy and triggered your brain into survival mode which caused you to become hyper focused at the task at hand. This is truly amazing.

Another reason you feel good and are hyper focused is because of ketone bodies. When you enter intermittent fasting you produce ketone bodies that is tremendous brain fuel. We also learned that when you are in ketosis you produce ketone bodies. You see how we can use the keto diet and intermittent fasting to our benefit.

What exactly do I mean by cellular benefits?

There is something in our body that is called autophagy which literally means self-eating. Autophagy is a detox process your body undergoes to clean out damaged cells and regenerate new ones. The protein that we must give a thank you to is p62 because that protein activates to induce autophagy. The newer cells that are built are stronger, more powerful, and more efficient. This will help your skin glow better which can boost self-esteem and how you view yourself. The best part of this autophagy is that you will have improved your organ function which has correlated to a longer life span. So basically, in an indirect way intermittent fasting can help you live longer. Okay enough benefits how do I start!

How do I start to intermittent fast?

What you eat leading into a fast makes all the difference. Eating a high fiber meal or snack before you start your fast will keep you full for a longer period. The struggle with intermittent fasting is the hunger you feel during the fast. If you are going to fast for 16 hours then I recommend that you eat a fiber meal or snack before you commence the fast. The high fiber meal can be very simple for example you could eat psyllium husk, broccoli, flaxseed, carrots, Brussels sprouts, oats, beans, lentils, and many other choices. This will help with the hunger problem associated with intermittent fasting. A healthy fat before the start of a fast will help you twofold. Fats digest slower which will keep you full for a longer time. Also, fats will leak fatty acids into your bloodstream so you can produce those ketone bodies we talked about. You could also eat some protein but the main concern is to get the fiber and fat right before the start of a fast. This will make all the difference and give you an edge on staying full longer. This can be as simple as eating broccoli with some coconut oil at night before you go to sleep. This will set you apart from other people who tried intermittent fasting and failed because they were too hungry.

How long should I fast?

This is up to you. Some people fast for 10 hours and work up to 20 hours. This is a good strategy to acclimate your body to the fast. The benefits increase the longer you fast. So, if you fast for a shorter time you will get more body composition or physical benefits. If you fast for a longer time you will increase the amount of cellular rejuvenation or autophagy effects the body goes under. I recommend you start off with a 16 hour fast if you are a beginner. This means you will not eat for 16 hours and you will have an 8-hour window to eat as much as you want. 16 hours is the bare minimum to see dramatic results. If you fast less than 16 hours you will be getting benefits but it is not exactly the true intermittent fasting benefits we talked about. Now the benefits increase exponentially every hour after 16 hours. If you can't start at 16 then start somewhere lower. The goal is to work your way up to 20 hours. I recommend that you start your fast at 10pm the night before and continue until 2pm the following day. This is perfect and easy because you can sleep for most of the fast. During 2pm to 8pm you can eat whatever you want. Since this is mostly a keto book I assume you want to eat keto meals which is perfect with this diet. I recommend eating the mixed spring green salad before starting your fast. You can add more food to the recipe if you would like but this is just an example of one of the recipes you could use.

Can I eat anything during the fast?

The answer is yes but it depends. I recommend you follow a true fast but there are a limited number of things you can consume. You can consume black coffee without any sweetener or creamer. Black coffee is very interesting because it will not break your fast and will actually speed up the process of the cells being recycled.

One study was published in the Journal Cell cycle speaking to this phenomenon. Polyphenols are compounds found in foods and they help protect against some health problems. The study showed that polyphenols in decaf or caffeinated coffee recycle cells and go through autophagy more than cells that were not exposed to coffee. This means that caffeine supports our fast. Coffee will help boost fast loss and support autophagy. Black coffee is truly amazing. If you add sugar to it your body at this point is very insulin sensitive and you will have an increase in insulin if you eat sugar during your fast. This will cause an increase in blood sugar levels and we don't want this so please stay away from sugars.

Another great source that will not break a fast is tea. Black tea or green tea is all fair game when fasting. Do not consume bulletproof tea or bulletproof coffee because that has sugar. Remember that sugar triggers a metabolic response for example the increase of insulin hormone in blood. I will hope to make a future book about the science behind these words we hear every day relating to our health. Also, if you were wondering water is 100 percent okay to consume.

What should I eat at the end of my fast?

I recommend looking at this by thinking of health. I recommend breaking a fast with a bone broth. This allows the collagen in the bone broth to restore the gut. When you fast you temporarily weaken the gut mucosal layer that protects you from acid or trauma in the gut. If you eat bone broth the gut can absorb things better. This will solve the issue of having an upset stomach after breaking a fast. So, about 8 ounces of bone broth at the end of a fast is enough to trigger this gut healthy benefit. Now listen closely for whatever reason do not mix fats and carbohydrates. Carbohydrates will cause an insulin spike which in simple terms will open the cell up. Now this is fine but the problem arises when you eat something high in carbs and high in fats. Since the cell is open when it gets a carbohydrate the fat will go into the cell as well. You don't want this to happen. We don't want our fats to go into ours cells they have a different way of being metabolized and we must respect that.

So, the golden rule is to never consume carbohydrates and fats at the same time. I'm talking about eating something high in carbs and high in fat for example eating pasta and an avocado at the same time. This would be very bad and if you do this personally then this may be a reason why you have not seen the best results with all the diet plans you have tried out.

You can eat an avocado alone and be fine but once you eat a high carb that is the issue.

Now, thankfully this is a book about keto and every single recipe has a very small margin of carbohydrates. So, pick and choose what you want to eat from all the recipes we have discussed. Overall, you can eat carbs and protein or fats and proteins.

When should I start my workout?

You can workout after you break your fast or during your fast. If you want to burn the most fat then you must train during your fasted state. Training during the fasting period will allow you to receive more physiological effects. The idea is if you workout right before you break your fast you will be able to burn the most fat possible because your metabolism is increased. Your body at this point is burning fat at a high rate because that is what research has proved with intermittent fasting. That is a fact. Now if we exercise during the fasted state we have in a sense sped up the process of burning fat. Now if you do choose to workout right at the end of your fasted state you will see some performance decline because your body is a little weaker.

Now if you workout right in the middle of your fast you will not see any performance decline because your body is not weakened by the fast yet. I recommend working out in the middle of your fast because you are not weakened by the fast and you can still receive the benefit from fasting.

Now you can also workout after you break your fast too. The only concern when doing this is not letting your body properly digest the food before you workout. When you ingest food to break a fast there is a lot of blood that will be pumping into your gut to digest the food. If you workout when you haven't fully digested then you are detracting from the gut. This means you are pumping blood away from the gut to the body part being used to perform the exercise at hand. When you do this you are not absorbing the nutrients the way you should be. So do not do this and work out a little bit later so you have fully digested everything.

What are the different types of fasting?

The first one is intermittent fasting. The second one is prolonged fasting. This fasting lasts all the way from 24 hours to 48 hours. This type of fast triggers more of the cellular rejuvenation benefits and mental benefits. Research has shown that the longer you fast the more your mental acuity sharpens. An important factor to consider is that after 48 hours the physiological body composition effects start to decline. You only want to do this once a month if you are interested in more cellular rejuvenation.

Another type of fast is called the liquid fast. This is where you can consume only liquids such as coffee, bone broth, bullet proof coffee, and water. There is no metabolic benefit to this fast but it does allow the digestive system to rest. Finally, the last type of fast is called dry fasting. This is where you don't consume any food or water. Now this type of fast is interesting because it pulls hydrogen from fat stores to make molecular water. The body now burns more fat because it has to take portion of the fat to make water. The hydrogen from the fat will combine with the oxygen we breathe to make this molecular water. Now this is very intense on the body and should only be done every 6 months if interested.

Is there a difference in fasting between a man and a woman?

The answer is yes but only slightly. Men have it easy and they can just jump right into fasting because they don't have some of the obstacles a woman will face. The only real concern with women fasting would be because the reproductive system will be sending more hunger signals to brain than a man would. This is because the body is in a fight mode. Other than that there has not been any more research with concerns about male vs female. The only true difference will be that females experience more hunger than males.

What are the most common concerns with intermittent fasting?

Everyone wants to know if you lose muscle when you fast. An article published in the journal of translational medicine proves that intermittent fasting versus not intermittent fasting but eating the same amount of calories ended up resulting with subjects burning more fat while preserving more muscle. The subjects built more muscle than the ones who didn't intermittent fast. This means that muscle preservation is high in intermittent fasting.

Will intermittent fasting slow down my metabolism and affect my thyroid? If you decrease your intake of calories per day then your metabolism will change. If you don't change the amount of calories you intake then your metabolism will not change. The thyroid is a little more complex to explain. A study in the European Journal of Endocrinology says that during the fast the thyroid function stays the same. The only thing that changes are the thyroid precursors. The thyroid precursors will start to decrease in number. This means that the production of the thyroid hormone would start to slow down but the actual thyroid hormone itself would not slow down. In other words, the machine that creates the thyroid will start to slow down. Now only the subjects ingested food the thyroid precursors started to increase. So the machine that creates the thyroid starts to go up. Basically, once you start eating everything starts to balance out. Another factor to consider is that the thyroid rejuvenates very quickly.

When should I take my supplements? This is an easy one. If the supplement has carbs or calories, it breaks a fast. If the supplement is a soft gel that has been suspended in oil that will break your fast because it has a caloric affect. You want to consume those calories after you have already eaten. If the supplement is a water soluble vitamin like a multivitamin such as vitamin C, you can take that during your fast. Now, I recommend you stay true to your fast and not eat anything. Also, another factor to consider is that sometimes it can be hard on the stomach when you consume those supplements.

Can I drink alcohol during the fast? When you consume a drink it converts alcohol to acetaldehyde which is very toxic to body. The toxin is so toxic it jumps ahead of any food inside the body. So, the body will prioritize the breakdown of alcohol instead of anything else. Let's remember that fat burning occurs in the liver. If the liver is prioritizing the breakdown of acetaldehyde then the fat burning slows down. We want to increase the amount of fat we burn. If we drink alcohol and slow down the process then why are we even going to intermittent fast.

Conclusion

The keto diet can be used with the intermittent fasting lifestyle. We have gone through many recipes that you can make at home. You don't have to jump right into the diet or right into the intermittent fasting. If you do so you will want to quit and never attempt to try again. The secret to doing any diet is slow progression. You want to slowly acclimate your body and taste buds to a totally different diet. You can start out by eating keto meals only twice a week and then work to a full 7-day cycle. Once you can eat keto meals every day and not hate yourself for it then you can add intermittent fasting in the same manner you added the keto meals. This type of diet is very powerful and it has the ability to cure many people from a horrid disease that plagues us called diabetes. There are over thousands of people who can say the keto diet has changed their life towards a longer and healthier life.

Resources

www.thenourishedcaveman.com
www.easylocarb.azurewebsites.net
www.ketodietapp.com

Thank you for your time.
We enjoyed making this book. Help us out by
following our twitter account @ Minerva_PS_Co

Message Us Questions
We want to hear from you. It will help us produce
higher quality books for the future.

Lastly, leave a customer review if you liked the
book. If you didn't then let us know what we can
improve on.

INTERMITTENT FASTING:

101 Guide to Transforming Your Lifestyle Through Diet to Achieve Extreme Weight Loss for Women and Beginners

Minerva Publishing Services & Company

INTERMITTENT FASTING

101 Guide
to Transforming
Your Lifestyle Through
Diet to Achieve Extreme
Weight Loss for
Women and
Beginners

MINERVA P.S. & CO

MINERVA PUBLISHING SERVICES & COMPANY

Preface

Welcome to "Intermittent Fasting: How to Transform Your Lifestyle Through Diet for Better Health and Extreme Weight Loss." In this book, we will help you to understand the principles behind intermittent fasting and how it can help you.

- If you've tried and failed at every diet fad out there.
- If you're fed up with never having any energy and always feeling tired.
- If you wish there was an easier way to get the body of your dreams without all the calorie counting or drinking endless protein shakes.

Then you are in the right place!

When following an intermittent fasting regime, you simply eat normal amounts of healthy food, but just in a much shorter time frame called the eating window. For example, you eat all of your meals within an 8-hour period each day while eating nothing for the remaining 16 hours.

You may think this sounds hard, but actually, most people find it very simple. Remember that you don't eat while you're sleeping, and this forms a large part of your fasting period.

One of the best reasons to use fasting to lose weight is that it actually helps your body use its fat reserves as fuel, which reduces your body fat.

Fasting shouldn't be looked at as a diet. In reality, it should be used as a permanent adjustment to the way you eat food, combined with eating healthy nutritious foods.

If you are unhappy with your body or your health and are constantly changing your diet without getting the results you are looking for, the intermittent fasting lifestyle may be exactly what you need. The most important part of any successful nutritional plan is having it pertain to your entire lifestyle. This book will not only teach you about the science and benefits of an intermittent lifestyle but will also assist you in reforming other parts of your lifestyle, including exercise, in order to help you achieve revolutionary results.

Fasting is not recommended for children (under 18), women who are pregnant or breastfeeding, people with eating disorders or anyone who has a medical condition unless they get the approval of their doctor or a medical professional.

Chapter 1.

What is Intermittent Fasting?

In recent years Intermittent Fasting has taken the dieting, health and fitness world by storm. The reason for the popularity of intermittent fasting is undoubtedly its simplicity, quick results and numerous health benefits.

Although you may have heard about intermittent fasting, you might still be left wondering what it is and how to do it, so let's take a closer look and find out.

The Principals of Intermittent Fasting

Intermittent fasting is quite simply and eating pattern that revolves on a cycle between times that you are eating and times you are not eating or fasting.

Although intermittent fasting doesn't, in principle, involve any form of food restriction, calorie counting or food group elimination, it is advisable to remember that for best results from intermittent fasting a healthy balanced diet should also be incorporated.

There are various "cycles" of intermittent fasting, which we will look at in more detail in the next chapter, but to give you a basic idea, it is usual for people to fast daily.

We all fast naturally when we sleep at night. During that time our body functions on the energy provided by our food intake the previous day and don't require any further food while we are sleeping. This is why the first meal of the day is called "Break*fast*" as we are breaking our overnight fast.

When you are practicing intermittent fasting, most people choose to extend this fasting period and not eat their first meal until later in the day, perhaps at lunchtime.

You may wonder how you would cope without eating breakfast but, in fact, adapting your body to intermittent fasting is fairly easy to achieve. It is common after the first week of fasting to have increased energy levels and not, as you might imagine, reduced ones.

Many people think that they would suffer from hunger, and although this can be true, to begin with, it soon passes as your body adapts to your new eating cycle.

While you are in a fasting period you cannot eat, but you can drink zero calorie drinks such as water, black coffee and tea, infusions or calorie-free beverages (although these commercial beverages are not recommended as they often contain ingredients that are very bad for your health).

The taking of supplements during your fast is generally permitted, providing they are calorie free.

Why You Should Fast

In truth, fasting isn't new at all. In fact, we have been doing it for thousands of years. Before modern times, when food has become an easily accessible commodity for most, it was often a great deal harder to come by. During the winter months, food could be very scarce and even eating a single meal a day was often not possible. In these times man feasted in times of plenty, but also often starved in times of hardship.

Some religions also advocate fasting as part of their faith, including Christianity, Buddhism, and Islam.

When we are sick, we instinctively fast, so, as you see, in reality, there is nothing unusual or unnatural about fasting at all.

Fasting changes many of our body's processes. It safeguards us during times of famine so that our bodies can continue to thrive. This is done through changes in our genes and hormone levels and also provokes changes to our cellular repair processes.

When we have undergone fasting, our blood glucose levels and insulin levels are significantly reduced. We also see increases in human growth hormone. This can help us in two ways; it can help us to lose weight, as it automatically reduces our calorie intake, and to use more fat for energy. It also gives us a range of metabolic health benefits.

Evidence suggests that regular intermittent fasting can increase longevity, protect us from diseases such as type II diabetes, cancer, heart disease, Alzheimer's and more besides.

For some people who have struggled with other diets, they find intermittent fasting is the perfect answer, it is straightforward and easy to do and it gives good results quickly.

Essentially, it's a perfect "life hack" making weight loss simpler, as well as giving other added health benefits. Not to mention the amount of time saved preparing meals, and money saved buying food.

Intermittent fasting is seen as being generally safe to do, provided it isn't taken to extremes. The food you do eat should be healthy, balanced and nutritious and you should still avoid foods that are not considered good for your health, including:

- Processed foods – items made from white flour (bread, cakes, biscuits, pasta), white rice, processed meats such as ham, salami or bacon
- Foods high in saturated fats should be kept to a minimum. Foods containing trans fats should never form part of the human diet
- Foods high in added sugar

A healthy diet should include:
- Unprocessed foods made from whole grains
- Unprocessed organic meat and fish
- Organic vegetables and fruit
- Foods with monosaturated or

- polyunsaturated fats particularly Omega 3
- Organic free-range eggs
- Pulses, nuts, and seeds
- Nut milks

To Summarize

Intermittent fasting is restricting the times of the day when you eat food. It is natural, easy to do and can save you time and money. It can benefit your overall health and help you to lose weight

Chapter 2.

Types of Intermittent Fasting

As we discovered in chapter one, intermittent fasting involves periods of fasting and periods of eating. There are several ways to do this, and depending on your reason for using intermittent fasting, it is a good idea to choose a way that seems to best suit your lifestyle and personality. By this I mean if you are someone who can be very dedicated to what they are doing one of the tougher regimes may suit, but if you find willpower is a big issue, you may wish to start with a softer approach.

These are some of the more popular intermittent fasting practices:

The Diet

This involves fasting for two days and eating normally for the remaining five.
On fasting days, you are only permitted to eat between 500 and 600 calories.

This diet first became popular a few years ago and was favored by people who were used to calorie counting.

You are required to decide which two days of the week you will fast in advance and these are not usually sequential. For example, you might decide to fast on a Monday and a Friday.

The problem with this diet is that although you are restricting calories for 2 days you aren't truly fasting, as you can eat the food that gives you the calories at any time of the day. This diet, although relatively easy to do, is not true intermittent fasting and is generally not sustainable.

Eat Stop Eat

This is where a fast of 24 hours once or twice a weekly is followed. This diet became popular due to its creator, fitness expert Brad Pilon.

In this regime, you are required to fast after eating your dinner and not eat again for another 24 hours. So, if for example you ate your dinner at 7:00 p.m. on a Friday evening and didn't eat again until 7:00 p.m. on Saturday evening then you will have fasted for 24 hours.

This fast cycle can also be done from lunch to lunch

or breakfast to breakfast, providing you have a full 24 hours of fasting in between.

Zero calorie beverages are permitted throughout the fast, but no food.

Regular meals should be eaten when you are not fasting.

The main issues with this approach are that to go cold turkey and eat nothing for a full 24 hours can be very difficult. You may also have blood sugar problems that can cause you to feel faint, particularly if you have a job that required physical activity.

Because the fast is only done once or twice a week your body doesn't have time to adapt to the fasting periods, so it is always a shock to the system each time.

It is possible to start with shorter fasts of between 14 or 16 hours and build up to the full 24, but the likelihood is you will be ravenous by the end of your fasting period and this negative association will prevent you from continuing for very long. It may also encourage you to binge eat.

Eat Every Other Day Fasting

This fasting regime is exactly as the name describes, eating one day and fasting the next in a continual cycle.

This particular diet has several versions, some which allow up to 500 calories to be consumed on fasting days and somewhere no food can be consumed on fasting days.

The latter method of no food during fasting days is definitely not recommended for beginners, and it still has the disadvantage of your system never fully adapting, because you are either in feast or famine. Due to the harshness of this, it is again difficult to continue for a prolonged period and will cause negative psychological associations.

You can, of course, adapt it to suit you and see what level of calorie intake you find acceptable on fasting days and keep to a healthy diet on non-fasting ones.

The Eating Window Method

This is probably the most commonly used and successful of intermittent fasting approaches. Following this eating plan, you are required to fast for a set number of hours per day and are only permitted to eat within a strict eating window.

For example, you may fast from after eating your evening meal that you finished at let's say 7:00 p.m. and not allow yourself to eat again until noon the next day, this is a 17 hour fast with a 7-hour eating window where you can eat lunch at mid-day and your evening meal at 6:30 p.m. in the evening.

Some people prefer to only eat one meal a day, although this can be pretty extreme and beginners would find it difficult to achieve. You can, however, adopt this method to suit you, but you will need a fasting period each day of around 14 hours for women and 16 hours for men (or more), to achieve the best results.

The best part about this method is that most of the fasting is done at night while you are sleeping and denying yourself breakfast is something your body quickly and easily adapts to.

If you want to lose weight rapidly you can also restrict your calorie intake to 1000 a day, or use it in combination with another eating approach such as the Ketogenic diet, which causes the body to use fat as energy instead of glucose.

The eating window method is well tolerated because the body can quickly adjust itself to the routine. It is, therefore, one of the most successful weight loss methods.

If you particularly like eating breakfast then you can change your fasting period and skip dinner instead so you eat your first meal at say 8:00 a.m. and your lunch by 1:00 p.m., giving you an eating window of 5 hours and a fasting period of 19 hours for example.

Drinking water and other zero calorie drinks are fine as it is important to maintain good hydration throughout the day.

A healthy balanced diet should be eaten during the eating window and you should actively avoid "junk" foods.

If you are after an easy to maintain diet, then this could be the best option for you.

The Warrior Diet

This diet isn't true fasting, as it promotes the eating of small amounts of raw vegetables or fruit before a huge meal at night. It entails spending most of your day fasting (or under eating) and is modeled on a warrior lifestyle, when warriors would be busy hunting, gathering or fighting during the day and would then return home to feast at night.

This was one of the first diets that included a form of fasting and it also relies on the food you consume to be along the lines of the paleo diet, in that it should be raw whole foods that have undergone no processing and still look as they would in nature.

To Summarize

The human body is well adapted to dealing with periods of fasting. In fact, it is probably the most natural form of eating for a human being.

The most successful regime for incorporating fasting into your daily life is one that the body can become accustomed to and just forms part of the natural cycle of eating. This is why the eating window method is the best tolerated along with the warrior diet. It isn't necessary to count calories with either of these options but simply requires that you eat healthy nutritious food.

Lots of people have achieved amazing results using these methods, although intermittent fasting still won't be to everyone's taste. It has been equally successful in both men and women, but may not be suitable for people with eating disorders, due to the risk of under eating and binging.

Chapter 3.

The Health Benefits of Intermittent Fasting

In recent years there much by way of scientific evaluations has been done in intermittent fasting. This has demonstrated that intermittent fasting has a broad range of impressive health benefits. Not only can it help you to lose weight by using fat as energy, but it can also help prevent disease.

Weight Loss

The vast majority of people who try intermittent fasting are using it to help them lose weight. This works in two ways, firstly by reducing the number of overall calories being consumed, and secondly by improving hormone function that promotes weight loss.

This is due to the lowering of insulin levels along with the increase of norepinephrine, which is a growth hormone. This combination increases the metabolic rate and causes body fat to be broken down and used for energy.

The benefit of this double action is that weight loss is being promoted from two sides of the equation. The calories you are using are being increased, and the calories you are consuming are being reduced.

Most individuals see weight loss of between 3% and 8% over a three to twenty-four week period. If you look at it from another perspective and measure your waist circumference to gauge the amount of harmful belly fat lost, it can range between 4% and 7% in the same period.

Reduces Insulin Resistance and Risk of Type 2 Diabetes

The instance of type 2 diabetes has shown a dramatic rise in recent years. This is thought to be mostly due to poor diet and the consumption of foods that cause insulin levels to become raised over long periods, causing firstly insulin resistance and eventually resulting in type 2 diabetes.

Our body's primary energy source is glucose, which we get from the food we eat. In recent times the amount of glucose-producing foods we consume has increased dramatically.

High carbohydrate processed foods are one of the biggest causes and include breakfast cereals, white bread, white pasta, white rice and products made with refined wheat flour such as cakes, cookies, and pastries. These foods are rapidly broken down into glucose in the body and the sheer volume that floods the system causes a big problem.

Having too much glucose in the bloodstream is bad news, and the body wants to use it up as fast as possible. To achieve this Insulin is released into the body, it helps it use up the glucose for energy and well as taking it to your liver, muscles and (if there is too much, which there usually is) your fat cells.

To give you the basic idea, insulin works by rushing around your body telling all the cells "Hey guys, look, there's lots of glucose here for you to use as energy!" At first, the cells respond and take in the glucose, but quickly they become full and don't want any more, so they start ignoring the message that the insulin is giving them. The body's reaction to this is to release more insulin to try to convince the cells to take the glucose. The insulin levels are raised higher and higher and over a period of time, you become insulin resistant. Eventually, this can lead to type 2 diabetes.

Intermittent fasting can reverse insulin resistance and reduce blood sugar levels, so avoiding type 2 diabetes and kidney damage.

Cells, Genes, and Hormones

Fasting causes your body to initiate a cellular repair process and changes hormone levels that allow body fat to be used as energy more easily.

This is what happens during fasting:

Insulin. The level of insulin in the blood drops significantly, allowing fat to be more easily used for energy.

Human Growth Hormone. The amount of human growth hormone circulating in the blood increases to up to 5 times the normal levels. This increase allows fat to be used as an energy source and muscle mass to be *increased*.

Cellular Repair. The cells of the body become more active, repairing themselves and eliminating waste materials.

Gene Expression. Due to the beneficial effects fasting has on gene expression and the function of hormones and cells, it is anticipated that intermittent fasting practices may not only protect against diseases but actually increase longevity.

Inflammation and Oxidative Stress

Many chronic diseases, as well as aging, can be promoted by oxidative stress. This is when free radicals, which are unstable molecules, interact with other important molecules such as proteins and even DNA, damaging them.

When combined with a diet that is high in antioxidant-rich foods, intermittent fasting may help your body be more resistant to oxidative stress.

Inflammation, which is a fundamental cause of many common diseases, can also be reduced by intermittent fasting.

A study published in the online issue 16 of Nature Medicine, describes how β-hydroxybutyrate inhibits a complex set of proteins known as inflammasome, particularly NLRP3. The inflammasome is responsible for driving inflammatory response in disorders such as type 2 diabetes, Alzheimer's disease, autoimmune diseases, atherosclerosis, and other autoinflammatory disorders.

Heart Health

The biggest killer in the world is currently heart disease. Intermittent fasting can improve many of the risk factors associated with heart disease, including LDL cholesterol levels, blood pressure, triglycerides, inflammation, and blood sugar levels. Making a useful way to help prevent the disease long term. This is particularly useful for people who have a family history of heart disease.

Unfortunately, because intermittent fasting is of no interest to the pharmaceutical industry (because they can't make money from it), very little study has been done on humans to ascertain the full effects that intermittent fasting can provide. To really understand the full potential a lot more human trials need to be done.

Cellular Repair

Cellular repair, known as autophagy, is stimulated by fasting. Autophagy is when all the dysfunctional and broken proteins that have accumulated within the cells over time are broken down and eliminated. Autophagy can help protect the body against diseases such as Alzheimer's and cancer.

Cancer

Another disease that seems to have become more prevalent in recent times is cancer.

Cancer is the uncontrolled growth of cells, as the cells auto-destruct mechanism stops functioning and they continue to grow unhindered.

It is thought that when the body is in a fasting state that cancer cells cannot simply "wait out" the fast in the same way as normal cells do. Because they are permanently stuck in "on" mode, they cannot find the nutrients they need to sustain them during a fast. The healthy cells are unaffected, as they simply hibernate during the fast, which cancer cells cannot do.
Fasting is also useful for cancer prevention, as it reduces insulin resistance that is linked to several cancers. It also causes autophagy, where the cells clean out all the garbage, making them healthier.

As with heart disease, insufficient studies have been conducted to show the full potential of intermittent fasting in humans. We are now reliant on individual health associations to initiate the types of studies that are required to further prove the evidence gained to date.

The metabolic boost that intermittent fasting provides isn't only good for the body, it is good for the brain as well.

Oxidative stress, inflammation, blood sugar levels and insulin resistance all have negative effects on brain health. Intermittent fasting has been shown to generate new nerve cells that benefit brain function.

A brain hormone, brain-derived neurotrophic factor (BDNF) is increased with intermittent fasting. Deficiency in this hormone has been linked to depression and other mental health problems.

As intermittent fasting can also help to lower blood pressure to normal levels, it is helpful in the prevention of strokes and heart attack.

Alzheimer's Disease

Alzheimer's is the most common neurodegenerative disease and it is incurable. Prevention is, therefore, most definitely the best approach.

Patient's with Alzheimer's can benefit and show significant improvements when following short daily fasts.

Because fasting stimulates cell cleansing it is

believed that it can help to prevent the occurrence of disease and maintain brain health.

Other neurological diseases such as Parkinson's and Huntington's may also be prevented or improved with intermittent fasting.

As with most other diseases, more scientific research on humans is required to show the full potential intermittent fasting could have

Longevity

Most of us want to live a long and healthy life, and intermittent fasting could be one of the keys to helping you achieve this.

Fasting has been shown to extend the lifespan of rats in the same way as continuous calorie restriction increases lifespan. It was shown in one study published in the Journal of Nutrition, Volume 31, Issue 3, 1 March 1946, Pages 363–375, that rats fasted every other day lived 83% longer than rats that did not fast.

Although more research is necessary on human subjects, intermittent fasting has shown to be greatly popular amongst the anti-aging crowd.

Due to the positive effects on health, it isn't difficult to understand how intermittent fasting can help with an increased lifespan.

Chapter 4

Misconceptions about Fasting

There are many "old wife's tales" surrounding eating, and we will look at some of them here.

Skipping Breakfast

Most of us will have had it drummed in from an early age that "Breakfast is the most important meal of the day" or "If you skip breakfast, you'll get fat" and other such nonsense. Although note here that eating breakfast is important for children and children do not tolerate fasting as well as adults do.

The reasoning behind this is, if you don't eat breakfast you'll become excessively hungry, and are more likely to give in to cravings and binge eating.

What we know is that eating breakfast is not essential in adults, and in controlled trials, there is no difference between people who do or do not eat breakfast regarding weight.

Lots of Small Meals Are Better For the Metabolism

It is a popular belief that by eating little and often you will help to increase your metabolic rate, and your body will, therefore, use more calories.

Our bodies do use energy all of the time, and the energy used to digest and absorb nutrients from the food we eat also uses small amounts of energy. The theory here is that by eating regular small meals your body will use up more of the energy provided by these meals to digest them than it would if you just eat three square meals a day.

Although this theory sounds as if it could work, it is not actually based on scientific fact, which stipulates it is the **total amount of calories** you consume each day that matter, regardless of how many meals those calories are eaten in. For example, if you ate three meals each containing 500 calories or 6 meals each containing 250 calories the net result would be the same.

Frequent Eating Controls Hunger

Some people are natural grazers and seem to have a need to constantly have something in their mouth.

For some, frequent meals reduced hunger cravings, while others say that it actually increase their level of hunger. The reasons for this are probably to do with what is being eating and the individual's metabolism.

At the end of the day, there is no consistent evidence to prove eating more often will reduce hunger or the number of calories an individual consumes.

Frequent Small Meals Help You Lose Weight

As we have seen in point 3 above, frequent meals neither boost your metabolism nor reduce hunger. In fact, frequent eating has absolutely zero effect on the energy balance ratio and will therefore also have no effect on weight loss.

The Brain Must Have a Continual Glucose Supple

It is true that the brain requires glucose to function as it is the fuel our brain uses. However, eating lots of carbs to provide us with this glucose is completely unnecessary and risks spiking our blood glucose levels and increases our chances of becoming insulin resistant.

The body has no difficulty in producing plenty of glucose from using a process known as gluconeogenesis. Although most of the time this isn't even necessary due to the glucose reserves you have stored in your liver in the form of glycogen.
Even people who have endured long periods of starvation and receive very little by way of carbohydrates can produce ketone bodies from fat. These ketone bodies provide the brain with energy and can reduce the amount of glucose it requires

We have evolved to do this because we would have been subjected, as many parts of the world still are, too long periods of famine. If we hadn't developed this ability to fuel our brains, we would have become extinct.

Some people suffer from a condition called hypoglycemia, which is low blood sugar. If you are one of these people then you should attempt intermittent fasting with caution and build up your body's tolerances gradually over time.

No matter what your physical condition, it is always highly advisable to discuss any diet plans you have with your doctor before commencing them.

Constant "grazing" is not normal behavior for a human. We aren't cows or sheep. We are much more closely aligned to carnivores and are designed to have periods of fasting.

Links have been made and there may be a correlation between the frequent intake of food and damage to health. It is possible that it could lead to liver stress and an increased instance of fatty liver disease. It may also increase the instance of colorectal cancer.

Fasting Forces Your Body Into Starvation Mode

Continued long term starvation or decrease in the number of calories being consumed daily will cause your body to go into a state of thermogenesis (starvation mode). This is to help keep you alive as long as possible by using as little of the available reserves of energy than is absolutely necessary. When you are in thermogenesis your body can reduce the number of calories it uses each day by hundreds and happens with almost every type of restrictive diet.

Short term fasts have been shown to temporarily **increase** your metabolic rate. This is caused by the significant increase of norepinephrine in the blood, which instructs fat cells to break down so they can be used for energy. This is why intermittent fasting works so effectively.

The Body Can Only Digest a Small Amount of Protein From Each Meal

Somewhere in the mists of time, it was suggested that the human body is only able to digest 30 grams of protein from every meal. For this reason, eating small high protein meals every two to three hours was necessary to gain maximum muscle mass.

There is <u>no</u> scientific evidence to back this up. It does not appear to matter whether you eat lots of small meals or less frequent larger ones. It is just down to the amount of total protein you consume and not the number of meals you spread it over.

Intermittent Fasting Causes Muscle Wasting

It is known that general dieting when you are restricting your calorific intake, can cause the body to use muscle for fuel. However, there is no evidence to show that this is any more prevalent with intermittent fasting.

Many bodybuilders use intermittent fasting precisely to maintain high muscle mass while lowering body fat.

Intermittent Fasting Damages Your Health

Although some people believe fasting to be harmful, there is no proof. On the contrary, there seem to be many health benefits gained by intermittent fasting. As we discovered in the previous chapter on the benefits of intermittent fasting, not only can it help us lose body fat and reduce weight, it can also improve our health by protecting us from disease and even extend our longevity.

Intermittent Fasting Causes Overeating

It is true that many diets can lead us to overeat or start a binging cycle that can be difficult to break. After you have fasted, it is natural to eat a little bit more than you would have done if you had not fasted. However, because you will be eating less overall (fewer meals), it is very unlikely that your calorie intake will be any higher.

Overall food intake is reduced, due to the fasting periods and the fasting also boosts the metabolism, reduces insulin levels, raises the norepinephrine levels and increased human growth hormone by up to five times. This effectively causes you to use up your fat reserves, not gain more.

Chapter 5

The Effects of Intermittent Fasting

Intermittent fasting, as we have already discovered, can have many positive effects. In this chapter, we are going to delve a little deeper and look at why this is.

Insulin and Type 2 Diabetes

Insulin is the true cause of obesity and type 2 diabetes. The question for avoiding these things shouldn't be "How do I reduce my calorie intake?" it should be "How do I reduce my Insulin levels?"

The few drugs that are able to lower insulin, come at a price. They are expensive and they can have some serious side effects. A diet that is low in sugar and refined carbs is helpful to some, but often it isn't enough. The real answer to this problem is, as if you didn't already know, intermittent fasting.

The fasting physiology I am going to outline here was written by Dr. George Cahill. He explains how fasting can help us make a gradual shift from using glucose for energy to using fat instead:

Stage 1.
The body at this point is using exogenous glucose for energy, which simply means glucose that is sourced from outside of the body and comes from the food we eat. As we start fasting the body runs out of this form of glucose and is forced into the next stage.

Stage 2.
The body is now using glycogen, which is glucose stored in the body. The majority of body tissues are still using glucose for energy, but the muscles, liver and fat cells have started to use fat.

Stage 3.
The muscles, liver and fat cells are now using fat exclusively for their energy needs.

Stage 4.
The glycogen stores have by this point run out. The liver and kidneys now have to use a process called gluconeogenesis to produce glucose that is required by the brain, red blood cells and the inner part of the kidney, called the renal medulla.

Stage 5
The brain has now shifted to using ketone bodies that come from the breaking down of fat. The red blood cells continue to use glucose produced by the liver and kidneys. The glucose in the blood is no longer from exogenous sources (the food we eat) but is made by the body called endogenous sources.

The fat being used is mostly triglycerides, a triglyceride is made from one glycerol and three fatty acids, hence the name.

As you can see, because the body is using its own fat supplies and not glucose for its primary energy source, the insulin and blood glucose levels remain low, but energy levels remain high. It is a total win.

How Fasting Affects the Body While Exercising

The majority of body tissues have the ability to use fatty acids as fuel and it is only the brain and red blood cells that require glucose, which the body makes by using fat. It is at this point that in reality the entire body is fueled by fat and not by sugar.

The effect of this is that the amount of free fatty acids in the blood plasma skyrockets from being almost undetectable when the body is using glucose for energy.

Beta-hydroxybutyrate and Acetoacetate are the Ketones produced to feed the brain. Their production also shows a sharp increase when fasting.

The triglycerides used as energy are broken down into their component 3 fatty acids and glycerol. The glycerol is sent to the liver and converted to glucose in a process called gluconeogenesis to feed the red blood cells and the renal medulla. **The fatty acids feed the body's energy requirements directly**.

As you can see, fasting doesn't actually starve the body and particularly the muscles of fuel as some people believe. The glucose is simply replaced by fats. The upside to this is that the body can sore a practically unlimited supply of fat, but it can only store a very small amount of glucose. This is why when you are using glucose for fuel, your energy levels can be something of a roller coaster, going from high to low very quickly.

When we are fasting regularly and our body has learned to use fat instead of glucose as its primary energy source, the brain is powered almost entirely on ketones.

Contrary to popular belief, this is completely normal and is the way our body was designed to work. Sometimes people confuse this with ketoacidosis, a condition often experienced by type 1 diabetics, where large numbers of ketones are produced even when blood glucose levels are very high. This is due to the lack of insulin and instead of being used for fuel, the ketones just build up which can be dangerous.

In a four day fast, the fatty acids can increase by 373% while the blood glucose can drop from 4.9 to 3.5. Beta-hydroxybutyrate one of the ketones used to power the brain can increase by up to a massive 2527%!

Over four days, there will be a continual increase in adrenalin. But it is, however, the norepinephrine that increases the most, while epinephrine levels remain quite stable. This adrenaline increases energy levels at all times, even when the body is in its resting state, the effect of this is that the metabolic rate is increased dramatically.

So, what does all of this tell us in a nutshell?
1. Adrenalin levels are increased, particularly when combined with regular exercise. The level of maximum oxygen intake (VO_2) is also slightly increased.

2. You recover from exercise faster and build muscle more quickly due to the increased levels of growth hormone.

3. You use up your fat supplies for fuel with fatty acid oxidation.

4. Insulin levels drop.

The net result, is a leaner, healthier body, with improved muscle definition.

Any adult can do this. It will cost you nothing, you don't have to count calories, buy expensive foods or supplements and you will even save time and money because the amount of food you eat is reduced.

Cell Cleansing - Autophagy

Fasting causes cellular cleansing, which is particularly beneficial to the brain. This is called autophagy and is, looking at it directly, where the body eats itself. This may sound alarming, but in reality, it is a good thing.

Autophagy is the body's way of cleansing itself so it can detoxify, repair and regenerate. Autophagy reduces inflammation, optimizes brain function and slows aging. It is also believed that autophagy can help with neuroplasticity and cognitive function, this is beneficial for many neural diseases such as Alzheimer's and Parkinson's.

Stress Reduction

Tests have shown that fasting improves not only cognitive function but can also improve resistance to stressful stimuli. The decreased inflammation in the brain increases neurotrophic factors such as growth neurons that improve learning and memory.

Because fasting causes challenges for the brain, it adapts itself and builds pathways that cope with stress. This has similar results to regular exercise, both of which increase the brain's protein production to promote growth and strengthen synapses and neuron connections. They both also stimulate nerve cell production in the hippocampus region to increase ketone levels to feed the brain. In turn, this increases the number of mitochondria found in the neurons which helps the neurons to maintain connections, improving learning ability, memory and reducing the stress response.

There are also some indications that the DNA repair of the nerve cells is improved with intermittent fasting, which could produce possible treatments for Dementia or Dystonia.

Interestingly this happens regardless or calorie intake. It is the fasting periods that matter.

Chapter 6.

Cheat Days: How to Plan Appropriately

If you are using intermittent fasting to lose weight then there may be times when your fasting regime is interrupted due to circumstances beyond your control. Don't panic, there are ways you can ensure this doesn't cause too much disruption. In fact, cheat days are a good thing as they can help prevent a slowing of their metabolism from a continual process of more calories being used than are being consumed.

A cheat day is a way of fooling the body into believing that it is getting enough calories, which cause an increase in the metabolic rate.

Dieting can also often cause reduced levels of leptin a thyroid hormone that is necessary for fat burning. Using a cheat day can restore leptin to normal levels.

Cheat days are often highly coveted by dieters because it means a break for sticking with the often-intense regime and also because most of us like to be just a little bit wicked every now and then!

Why Cheat Days Work Well With Intermittent Fasting

Because you're naturally consuming fewer calories while fasting, due to the small eating window, it is actually quite hard to overdo the calorie intake even when you do cheat.

A typical meal of 1000 calories allows you to eat a cheat meal without necessarily going over your total daily calorie target, and even if you do, it is unlikely to be by much.

What's good about this, is that it doesn't risk much in the way of weight gain, providing you schedule the cheat meal to co-inside with your eating window.

Here's what you should do:
1. Plan your cheat meal to be within your normal fasting eating window.

2. Do a high-rep workout shortly before or after the meal so your body uses the additional glucose calories you consume.

3. Enjoy the freedom of being able to eat what you want, but don't binge!

4. After you've eaten your cheat meal, return to your normal fasting patterns and foods. Eating lots of carbs – even refined ones is not a big issue for a binge meal. They will spike your insulin levels and this, in turn, will cause glucose to be driven into your muscle tissues. If you've done a big workout just before the muscles will use most of this by turning it to muscle glycogen and it will cause very little by way of weight increase or fat gain.

Leptin

As I mentioned at the start of the chapter, it is possible to become deprived of the hormone Leptin when on a strict diet of any kind. By restricting calorie intake, the metabolic rate can slow down and having occasional cheat days can help to prevent this. Cheat days will increase leptin levels to normal concentrations and result in a faster metabolic rate.

Cheat days will depend on the goals you set for yourself. If fat loss is your main aim then planning a cheat day as often as once a week or as infrequently as once every three weeks should maintain the results you require. Cheating, if it is properly planned, can actually be beneficial.

Planning is the key to successful cheating. It can be easy if you have a bad day to just throw in the towel and let your emotions take over. This can, unfortunately, result in your eating every bit of sweet, high calorie, unhealthy food you can lay your hands on. This is one of the reasons why meal planning is really important. Knowing what you are going to eat and when makes it much easier to stay on track.

By planning your cheat day meals in advance, you also have some of your favorite treats to look forward, but can also maintain control. This can help to make weight loss a lot more pleasant.

Be reminded, however, that cheat days are not how you should be eating every day, they are AT MOST to be done one time per week. It can often be best to schedule them to be the same day each week, so there is no risk of "confusion."

Intermittent fasting isn't a diet, it is a way of eating. For optimum results, this should become the way you eat – period.

Remember this, DIETS DO NOT WORK in the long term – I will repeat, DIETS DO NOT WORK. Changing your eating habits FOR LIFE do.

Diets don't work because you will always return to your own bad habits when you finish your diet. You will not only regain the weight you lost but more weight besides. The only way to become healthy and keep weight off permanently is to make a permanent change to the way you eat.

Chapter 7.

Exercise and Intermittent Fasting

It is difficult to know when the best time to exercise is when you are using intermittent fasting. Most advice seems to point to exercising immediately before or after a meal is best, especially for anyone suffering from type 2 diabetes or metabolic syndrome.

Exercising when fasting may be good because the chances are your stored carbohydrates (glycogen) will probably be fairly depleted and exercise will deplete them further and help you start using fat as s fuel source instead.

The biggest problem with exercising when you are in a fasted state is that it increases the risk of your body breaking down muscle for fuel. You are also a lot more likely to run out of energy quicker.

If you repeatedly work out when fasting, it may cause your metabolism to slow down and your performance levels to drop.

So, what can you do to avoid these issues?

The success of any exercise or weight loss program depends on how effective, safe and sustainable it is over time. If you want to reduce your body fat and increase or maintain your fitness level then you need to know how to do it safely.

When to Eat

If you are planning to do a moderate to high-intensity workout then you should aim to do it shortly after eating a meal. This will help your body tap the energy it needs to work at optimum levels.

Hydration

Drinking water is critically important when fasting as it helps clear your body of toxins and hydrates every cell in your body. It is also needed to maintain body temperature, lubricate your joints and keep you healthy.

Electrolytes

Electrolytes are electrically charged salts that carry either a positive or negative charge.

The electrolytes we need most for the body are:
- Sodium (positive) Na+
- Potassium (positive) K+

- Chloride (negative) Cl^-
- Calcium (positive) Ca^{2+}
- Magnesium (positive) Mg^{2+}
- Bicarbonate (negative) HCO_3^-
- Phosphate (negative)PO_4^{2-}
- Sulfate (negative) SO_4^{2-}

Electrolytes are necessary to maintain the voltage across your cell membranes and to carry electrical impulses between nerves and to contract muscles.

The electrolyte concentrations in your blood are managed by the kidneys. When you do a big workout, you will naturally lose electrolytes, particularly potassium and sodium, in your sweat. It is important to replace these lost electrolytes and this can be done by using something like coconut water, which is low in calories and doesn't contain added sugars, unlike most sports drinks.

Dizziness

It isn't uncommon to feel dizzy if you push yourself too hard. Especially if you are exercising after a fasting period and haven't yet eaten. This is caused by low blood sugar or dehydration. Ensure you listen to your body and only push yourself as far as is comfortable.

Macros

Macros are the percentages of the food groups you eat split between carbohydrates, fats, and proteins.

- Carbohydrates provide 4 calories per gram
- Fat provides 9 calories per gram
- Protein provides 4 calories per gram

If you are doing strength workouts you will need to eat more unrefined carbohydrates on the day of your workout. If you are doing HIIT (High-intensity Interval Training) then you won't need so many carbs. Remember to avoid refined carbohydrates such as cookies, white bread or white pasta and so on.

If you are working out to body sculpt, you should eat high-quality protein after the workout to aid muscle regeneration. While strength training, you should eat around 20 grams of high-quality protein with complex carbohydrates within 30 minutes of finishing your workout.

Exercise for Body Type

There are three body types, Ectomorph, Mesomorph, and Endomorph. Not only do these body types describe how a person looks, but they also help us understand the best forms of exercise to use and the different metabolic factors that influence weight gain and loss between the types.

By understanding your specific body type, you will be able to successfully plan your diet and training regimen.

The right nutrition and exercise can completely change your appearance, regardless of body type.

Ectomorphs

People with this body type are often able to overeat, without gaining extra weight. They have a fast metabolism, which helps them stay resistant to weight gain.

The best type of exercise for an ectomorph is short and intense, with the main focus being on working the large muscle groups.

Ectomorphs have the ability to lose fat easily.

Ectomorph Characteristics:
- Slight bone structure, with a delicate frame
- Flat chested
- Small shouldered
- Lean muscled

- Thin
- Have difficulty gaining weight
- Fast metabolism

It can be difficult for ectomorphs to gain muscle mass. Due to their high metabolism and ability to use calories quickly and efficiently, they are better suited to eating a diet that is quite high in carbohydrates. For best results, these should be eaten just before or just after a workout. These should include plenty of fresh vegetables and fruit, some unprocessed starch whole grains.

High-quality protein and fat sources in the form of unprocessed meat, fish, eggs as well as vegetable sources such as lentils, beans, nuts, and seeds.

In order for an ectomorph to gain muscle mass, they would need to do targeted workouts and may require the help of a high-calorie weight gainer, in the form of shakes, which can help.

Ectomorphs can easily tolerate eating junk food on cheat days, but attention should be paid to getting enough protein.

Strength training incorporating a limited amount of cardio is best. Using routines that involve heavy compound movements with minimal isolation for individual muscle groups (heavy weights, low repetition). Supersets can also be beneficial. Carbing up before and after exercise can prevent too many calories being burned.

Mesomorphs

Sporting an athletic body, with medium bone structure and strong lean muscle mass, the mesomorph is the best body type of those wanting to do bodybuilding and high muscle sporting activities.

Mesomorphs run testosterone high and are often growth hormone dominant. This predisposition aids in muscle gain while maintaining a low body fat ratio.

It is necessary for mesomorphs to maintain better control of their calorie intake as they can gain excess body fat more easily than ectomorphs.

A combination of weight training and cardio is best for body sculpting for those with a mesomorph body type.

Mesomorph Characteristics:
- Athletic build
- Usually hard bodied
- Strong well-defined muscles

- A rectangular body shape with a small waist and hips with broad shoulders
- Find gaining muscle easy
- Can tend to gain excess fat more easily than ectomorphs

Food
A mixed diet of balanced unrefined carbohydrates and high-quality proteins and fats with a macronutrient split of 40% carbs, 30% protein and 30% fat are good for mesomorphs.

A nutritious diet is essential if gaining body mass without fat is desired. To gain the best strong lean muscle foods such as eggs, poultry, seafood, kefir, Greek yogurt, green vegetables, beans, and whole grains can be beneficial.

Most mesomorphs have a reasonable carbohydrate tolerance, so meals that are carb heavy can be tolerated before and after a workout.

Other beneficial foods include fruits, nuts, and seeds.

Training
Mesomorphs tend to be naturally strong and their bodies respond fast to exercise. Regular resistance training with moderate to heavy weights can help build muscle mass. HIIT and compound body exercises in two to three sets of eight to 12

repetitions with a 30 to 90-second rest between sets are also beneficial.

Endomorphs

With the highest total body mass and a tendency to carry extra fat, along with the largest bone structure, endomorphs tend to be rather on the heavy side.

Endomorphs have a solid, but soft body that gains fat easily. They tend to be shorter and stockier with thick arms and legs.

They have strong muscles, particularly in the upper legs and are good for lifting very heavy weights for short period (deadlifts), or playing in defensive positions in sports.

Endomorphs then to be insulin dominant and have a low carbohydrate tolerance.

Exercise is an important part of the daily routine for an endomorph, they often suffer from a sluggish metabolism, but if educated to eat the right foods and do the right exercise they can maintain a strong, powerful physique.

Endomorph Characteristics:
- Rounded body shape
- Gains fat easily

- Gains muscle easily although it is often undefined
- Usually short and stocky in build
- Finds fat loss difficult
- Generally slow metabolism

Food

Endomorphs should stay away from carbs and ideally work on a macronutrient intake of 25% carbs, 35% protein, and 40% fat. Using a Ketogenic eating style combined with intermittent fasting gives the best results for this body type and it should learn to fuel itself from fat rather than carbs.

All carbs eaten should be dense unrefined carbs including whole grains, quinoa, millet, oats, sweet potatoes, nuts, and seeds.

Training
To reduce fat gain endomorphs, need to use high cardio exercise as well as high repetition weights (low weight high repetition) to maintain a streamlined physique and burn the most fat. Typically, endomorphs should train four or more times per week aiming to increase muscle mass and metabolic rate.

For best results endomorphs should:
- Train for a minimum of 20-minutes each day

- Work the larger muscle groups such as the legs and back
- Choose exercise that requires continuous rhythmic movement such as running, cycling or power walking, and not ones where there is a lot of starting and stopping, such as HIIT or tennis
- Choose an exercise regime that requires moderate intensity

Exercise Types

Whatever type of exercise you choose, ensure that you build it up gradually to avoid overdoing things and putting yourself off, or worse, causing yourself an injury.

Try to choose an exercise that you find enjoyable as it will be much easier to continue long-term. If you find you're not enjoying something, then find something else you do like, don't just stop exercising.

There are different types of exercise:
Low Impact
- **Power walking** – this is no gentle stroll in the park, but a purposeful walk that raises heart rate and even makes you break a sweat

- **Cycling, mountain biking or spinning** – getting in the saddle can help your leg strength and aerobic fitness, working your heart and lungs
- **Gym machines** – Cross-trainer, elliptical machine, ski machine, rowing machine or stepper.
- **Swimming** – there is more to do in the pool than just swim, there are various classes you can try out too, water aerobics, paddle boarding, spinning – yes that really is cycling in the water and more. Check out what's available at your local pool
- **Low impact exercise classes** – talk to the instructor

High Impact
- **Jump rope** – getting out the skipping rope and honing your skills is a great way to boost leg strength and aerobic fitness levels, it also makes you light on your feet
- **Running** – start off with a gentle jog, but as your fitness levels grow, add some sprints, hill work, and steps to really notch it up a level or two
- **CrossFit** – this is a training program designed to work around anyone regardless of fitness level, age or gender. It combines many kinds of exercise with nutrition. Find a group near you

- **P90X** – this is an intense workout program that you can do at home using the DVDs. You will also require additional equipment such as a pull-up bar, dumbbells, resistance bands, and an exercise mat. The program requires you to work out for 1 to 1.5 hours per day and also includes a nutrition program. You are required to take a fitness test before starting P90X and it isn't suitable for the unfit

- **HIIT** – High-intensity interval training. This type of workout combines short burst of intense activity with short rest periods. The idea is to work to your maximum capacity for the active periods so you really push yourself to the limit. The workouts are typically around 30 minutes and are suitable for any fitness level. HIIT workout can use running, swimming, cycling, strength training and exercise movements such as squats and push-ups.

Stretch Exercise

Yoga, Pilates, and Tai Chi are all forms of stretching exercise. They improve your suppleness and are useful for fine body sculpting. While the intensity level of these forms of exercise is not generally sufficient for using fat. This type of exercise should form part of your weekly routine, but it is the cardio work that will really help you to lose most fat.

Remember that you should always aim to eat shortly before or just after you exercise. This helps your body to burn calories more efficiently and will give you the best results.

Conclusion

Fasting is easy to do. It is simply a matter of eating to a schedule and can be as simple as cutting out food for a specified number of hours per day (not eating from your final evening meal at 7:00 p.m. until 1:00 p.m. in the afternoon of the following day).

Intermittent fasting can help you to lose weight by causing your body to use fat for fuel instead of glucose.

Intermittent fasting can help to prevent diseases such as diabetes, heart attack, stroke, cancer, Alzheimer's and Parkinson's and could even extend your lifespan.

Insulin resistance can be reversed by intermittent fasting.

There are many misconceptions about fasting, most of these are incorrect or only partially correct. By fasting correctly and using planned cheat days you can be sure that you get the best possible results from fasting.

Fasting is beneficial in other ways too. Not only will it help you to lose weight in the form of fat, but it also speeds up your metabolism, balances blood sugar levels (helping you sustain energy throughout the day) and best of all, it causes autophagy (cell cleansing).

No matter what body type you have intermittent fasting can have positive effects, especially when combined with correct exercise and nutrition.

Intermittent fasting can:
- Help you lose weight

- Assist in rebalancing your hormones

- Decrease insulin levels

- Reverse insulin resistance

- Help prevent diseases such as diabetes, Alzheimer's, heart disease and cancer

- Improve brain function

- Reduce stress response

Intermittent fasting is suitable for adults, regardless of age or fitness level. It is not suitable for children, pregnant or breastfeeding women or people with eating disorders. You should discuss any form of weight loss protocol with your doctor or health professional before starting.

We hope you have enjoyed reading this book and that it has helped you to understand and follow an informed intermittent fasting protocol. We wish you the best of luck in achieving the body of your dreams along with excellent health and longevity.

References

https://www.healthline.com/nutrition/what-is-intermittent-fasting

https://www.healthline.com/nutrition/intermittent-fasting-guide#methods

https://www.healthline.com/nutrition/11-myths-fasting-and-meal-frequency

https://news.yale.edu/2015/02/16/anti-inflammatory-mechanism-dieting-and-fasting-revealed

https://www.nature.com/articles/nm.3804#

https://hope4cancer.com/blog/healing-cancer-on-time-how-intermittent-fasting-may-help/

https://idmprogram.com/fasting-and-lipolysis-part-4/

https://health.howstuffworks.com/wellness/diet-fitness/information/question565.htm

https://www.smartdietandnutrition.com/intermittent-fasting-cheat-day-6-tips-to-success/

http://healthandstyle.com/body-type/exercise-for-endomorphs/

https://www.ncbi.nlm.nih.gov/pubmed/24440038

https://www.ncbi.nlm.nih.gov/pubmed/10837292

https://www.ncbi.nlm.nih.gov/pmc/articles/PMC2622429/

https://www.healthline.com/nutrition/10-health-benefits-of-intermittent-fasting

https://www.healthline.com/health/how-to-exercise-safely-intermittent-fasting

http://thescienceofeating.com/food-combining-how-it-works/workouts-for-all-areas/the-3-body-types-explained/